A Handbook of
Obstetrics and Gynaecology

A Handbook
of Obstetrics
and Gynaecology

A Guide for Housemen

R. S. Ledward BSc, MPS, MRCS, LRCP,
DA, DHMSA, MRSH, DM, FRCS, FRCOG

Consultant Obstetrician and Gynaecologist
William Harvey Hospital, Ashford, Kent,
South East Kent Health District, UK

Previously Fellow in Anesthesiology,
University of Virginia, Charlottesville, USA
Visiting Professor in Obstetrics and Gynecology,
Rutgers Medical School, New Brunswick,
New Jersey, USA

With a Foreword by
Professor E. M. Symonds

WRIGHT
Bristol
1986

Published under the Wright imprint by
IOP Publishing Limited
Techno House, Redcliffe Way, Bristol BS1 6NX

British Library Cataloguing in Publication Data
Ledward, R.S.
   A handbook of obstetrics & gynaecology.
   1. Gynecology   2. Obstetrics
   I. Title
   618   RG101

ISBN 0-7236-0848-2

Typeset by
BC Typesetting
51 School Road, Oldland Common, Bristol BS15 6PJ

Printed in Great Britain by
The Bath Press, Lower Bristol Road, Bath BA2 3BL

PREFACE

It is not intended for this book to provide all the answers to all the problems encountered in obstetrics and gynaecology—no such book has been written. It is designed as a discussion document to encourage teaching seminars between student, resident or general practitioner with the consultant in the local hospital. Many, if not most, obstetricians differ in their approach to a particular problem—the management of pregnancy-induced hypertension is *par excellence* an example of the various regimes available and which appear fashionable in various centres throughout the country and the world, e.g. chlormethiazole may be selected as the drug of choice in Scotland; hydrallazine and diazepam in England, whilst in Dallas, USA, magnesium sulphate will be first-line therapy. The alternative approaches mentioned in the book will hopefully form the basis for discussion.

Cross reference between various sections throughout the book is given, further reading is encouraged and a suggested bibliography is provided.

It is hoped that students reading for the final MB, ChB or diploma examination of the Royal College of Obstetricians and Gynaecologists will find it of value and that it will also be of value for midwives and general practitioners.

R. S. Ledward, 1986
South East Kent Health Authority

ACKNOWLEDGEMENTS

The preparation of this manuscript has only been made possible by the most valuable help provided by colleagues from other disciplines and my grateful thanks are extended to all who have helped with their appropriate contributions.

I wish also to thank those who read the manuscript—both at senior and junior level—who have made constructive improvements.

Finally, I am extremely grateful to Mrs Jean Gipson for her patience in typing the manuscript and to Mr Roy Baker of my publishers for his kind help.

The following figures appear in this book by courtesy of the indicated organizations:

Fig. 2.1 is reproduced with the permission of
Scientific and Industrial Equipment (Reading) Ltd (SIEL).

Fig. 3.2 is reproduced with the permission of
Portex Ltd, Hythe, Kent.

Figs 5.4–5.6 are reproduced with permission of Mr P. Steer (Editor) *Fetal Heart Rate Patterns and their Clinical Interpretation* and of Sonicaid Ltd, Chichester, W. Sussex.

Figs 5.7, 5.8, 8.1, 8.2 are reproduced with the permission of Rocket of London Ltd, Watford.

Fig. 6.1 is reproduced with the permission of
Seward Medical, London.

Figs 10.1 and 10.2 are reproduced with the permission of Ethicon Ltd, Scotland and *The Digest of Obstetrical and Gynaecological Procedures* (1980).

Fig. 12.2 is reproduced with the permission of
Spembley Medical Ltd, Andover, Hampshire.

Rodney S. Ledward, 1986
South East Kent Health Authority

CONTENTS

Abbreviations		ix
Definitions		x
Personal management of cases		x
Foreword		xi
Part I	**Obstetrics**	1
1	Pre-pregnancy clinics	3
2	Associated medical and surgical disorders	9
3	Antenatal clinics	19
4	Antenatal wards	31
5	Fetal monitoring	35
6	The labour ward	51
7	General practitioner obstetric units	73
8	Obstetric analgesia and anaesthesia	80
9	The postnatal ward	90
10	Surgical procedures	98
Part II	**Neonatology**	109
11	Neonatology: Special care baby unit	111
Part III	**Gynaecology**	117
12	Out-patient clinics	119
13	Abortion	129
14	Infertility	140
15	Cytology, colposcopy and histopathology	149
16	Haematology	154
17	Clinical chemistry	159
18	Microbiology	165
19	Radiotherapy and oncology	174
20	Radiology and ultrasonography	183
21	Gynaecological surgery	189
22	Pharmaceutical services	198
23	Clinical budgeting	207

Appendices

I	Weight conversion chart	213
II	Supraregional assay service	214
III	Postgraduate training and examinations	216
IV	Emergency obstetric service ('Flying Squad' equipment)	220
V	Postmortem examinations	223
VI	Stillbirths	228
VII	Guidelines for the training of male student nurses	229
VIII	Useful telephone numbers	230

Index   233

ABBREVIATIONS

APH	antepartum haemorrhage
ARM	artificial rupture of membranes
BPD	biparietal diameter
C & S	culture and sensitivity
DRCOG	Diploma of the Royal College of Obstetricians and Gynaecologists
DVT	deep vein thrombosis
ECV	external cephalic version
FBS	fetal blood sample
FH	fetal heart
FHR	fetal heart rate
FPC	family planning clinic
FRCS	Fellow of the Royal College of Surgeons of England
GA	general anaesthetic
GP	general practitioner
LBW	low birth weight
LMP	last menstrual period
MRCOG	Member of the Royal College of Obstetricians and Gynaecologists, London
MRCP	Member of the Royal College of Physicians, London
MSU	mid-stream specimen of urine
PE	pre-eclampsia
PPH	postpartum haemorrhage
RMO	resident medical officer (house officer, senior house officer, intern)
SHO	senior house officer
SFD	small for dates
TB	tuberculosis
VDRL } TPHA } WR }	abbreviations for serological tests for syphilis

Definitions
1. Throughout this text the word *husband* covers the over-all term of 'accepting husband' or 'significant other'.
2. The terminology appertaining to *staff* relates to the male gender, but the text applies to either sex.
3. '*Bed rest*' implies almost total bed rest though the patient is allowed up to the shower and lavatory.

Personal Management of Cases
Each case should be managed according to the personal edict of the consultant under whom the patient is admitted. At night and weekends the management will be ordered by the consultant on duty. Patients admitted as an 'emergency' should be admitted under the consultant on duty unless the admitting condition relates to an acute on chronic condition when the patient should be admitted under whichever consultant she attended previously with that condition.

FOREWORD

by Professor E. M. Symonds MD, FRCOG
Department of Obstetrics and Gynaecology,
Queen's Medical Centre, University of Nottingham, UK

Every medical student is subjected to a barrage of information during his medical course. Having graduated from
the comforts and support of the experienced medical
teachers, the newly fledged doctor has now to face up to the
challenges of accepting clinical responsibility and initiating
positive, practical manoeuvres. Rodney Ledward has
clearly remembered his residency in obstetrics and
gynaecology and has compiled a book which provides
strictly practical guidelines for day-to-day management in
obstetric and gynaecological wards. This book is a
practitioner's guide to the clinical and practical aspects of
obstetrics and gynaecology and provides ready access to
information in the management of events that commonly
present to the new clinician—the new Resident or even
the General Practitioner with an Obstetric and Gynaecological interest. I am sure it will provide a useful and helpful
reference source for the resident staff, and act as a teaching
manual between junior and senior members of staff.
Mr Ledward compiled such information when he was
Senior Registrar and Clinical Tutor at the University of
Nottingham and he has expanded this format to provide
this valuable addition to guidelines for clinical practice.

PART I

Obstetrics

Chapter 1

Pre-pregnancy Clinics

INTRODUCTION

In every sophisticated community, patients should now be encouraged to attend their general practitioner for pre-pregnancy counselling. This particular area of constructive advice overlaps many other areas of medicine and, for the well-motivated woman, there is little need for anxiety; however, for other patients with medical disorders stricter guidance is required. Advice is necessary for all patients who may be planning a pregnancy within the near future and all responsible members of the community should be alert to encouraging their associates to accept professional advice.

Those involved with pre-pregnancy counselling include the general practitioner and appropriate hospital colleagues, family planning clinics, infertility clinic counsellors, health education workers, teachers of human reproduction, community midwives, health visitors, media propaganda staff through the Central Office of Information and the Health Education Council, the pharmacist (from whom the patient may purchase non-prescription medicines) and ultimately the patient herself.

The basic principle remains:

> 'All women in the reproductive years should be considered to be pregnant or potentially pregnant unless proved otherwise'.

COUNSELLING

Special pre-pregnancy clinics have been established in various centres, but many general practitioners will initiate their own counselling advice centre with appropriate referral to specific specialists. Advice covered includes the standard therapeutic format for all conditions:

Hospital or Home

The patient may wish to discuss with her own practitioner the merits of hospital or home delivery.

Nursing Care

Appropriate nursing care will be provided and explained to the patient.

Diet

Many patients will be outside the limits of normal weight (*Table* 1.1) as provided by the life insurance companies and advice regarding sensible diet and exercise should be provided.

Psychotherapy

Explanation of any investigation or therapeutic measures prior to conception should be provided; advice regarding antenatal screening techniques may be appropriate and encouragement to book early in their pregnancy and to attend antenatal booking clinics. The pre-pregnancy clinic will provide an opportunity for further discussion on past obstetric performance such as an unexplained stillbirth. Referral to specialized genetic counselling departments may be indicated.

Where patients are at risk for a sex-linked disorder, inborn error of metabolism or translocation carrier, preconception counselling will include a discussion on the possibility of first trimester prenatal diagnosis by chorion biopsy or amniocentesis at sixteen weeks' gestation.

Table 1.1. Normal weight table with upper and lower accepted weight limits

Height in shoes		Weight in indoor clothes 'Norm'				Height in shoes		Weight in indoor clothes 'Norm'			
ft	ins	stones	lbs	stones	lbs	ft	ins	stones	lbs	stones	lbs
4	8	6 / 9	6 / 12	8	8	5	8	8 / 13	10 / 4	11	8
4	9	6 / 10	8 / 1	8	11	5	9	8 / 13	13 / 9	11	12
4	10	6 / 10	11 / 5	9	0	5	10	9 / 14	2 / 0	12	2
4	11	6 / 10	13 / 8	9	3	5	11	9 / 14	5 / 5	12	7
5	0	7 / 10	1 / 12	9	6	6	0	9 / 14	9 / 11	12	12
5	1	7 / 11	3 / 1	9	9	6	1	9 / 15	12 / 2	13	2
5	2	7 / 11	6 / 5	9	12	6	2	10 / 15	2 / 7	13	7
5	3	7 / 11	9 / 9	10	2	6	3	10 / 16	6 / 0	13	13
5	4	7 / 12	12 / 0	10	6	6	4	10 / 16	10 / 6	14	14
5	5	8 / 12	1 / 5	10	10	6	5	11 / 16	1 / 13	14	10
5	6	8 / 12	4 / 9	11	0	6	6	11 / 17	5 / 6	15	2
5	7	8 / 13	7 / 0	11	4						

See Appendix I for conversion to kg.

Many patients may have had a previous termination of pregnancy and require assurance about their possibility of future conception. Other patients may be relatively infertile and require appropriate advice.

INVESTIGATIONS

Appropriate investigations in addition to routine weight and blood pressure assessment include:

1. Haemoglobin, blood grouping, serological tests for syphilis, urinalysis for culture and sensitivity.
2. Haemoglobin electrophoresis, sickle-cell screen.
3. Assessment of rubella status.
4. Karyotyping of both partners if any family history indicates the need for genetic assessment.
5. Stool for ova in recently arrived immigrants. Chest radiograph where indicated, especially in recently arrived immigrants.
6. Assessment of medical disorders—diabetes mellitus, thyroid dysfunction, hypertension and renal disease.

SURGERY

Surgery may be indicated for thyroid dysfunction uncontrolled by medical therapy; advice as to the wisdom of insertion of a cervical suture (annular suture) prior to conception may be sought.

DRUGS IN PREGNANCY

For a review of drugs in pregnancy *see* Ledward and Hawkins (1983). There is little place for drug therapy at the pre-pregnancy clinic but epileptic patients on therapy may benefit from folic acid in addition to their anti-epileptic treatment. Patients having long-term treatment with immunosuppressive or anticoagulation drugs, or anti-convulsants could have their regimen modified. Vitamin supplementation may help to reduce the incidence of neural tube defects (Smithell *et al.*, 1980).

More importantly, it is essential to stress the hazards of medication in and prior to conception and pregnancy. Many patients may require and receive tetracycline for acne, subsequently conceive and request a termination of pregnancy. Patients may attend for pre-pregnancy counsel-ling when their primary aim is initially appropriate contraception. Similarly the pre-pregnancy clinic would be an appropriate time to offer advice regarding the dis-continuation of drugs of addiction, including cigarettes, alcohol and drugs of abuse.

Summary

All women planning a pregnancy should preferably consult their general practitioner prior to conception for appro-priate advice and specific investigations. Practitioners should enquire as to the possibility of pregnancy prior to treating any condition with drugs or undertaking investi-gations harmful to pregnancy, e.g. intravenous urography.

RUBELLA VACCINATION

Rubella vaccination should be arranged where indicated.

CONTRACEPTION

This subject should be mentioned during the antenatal period. The subject is extensive and the reader is referred to the bibliography for a full review (Hawkins and Elder, 1979).

FURTHER READING

Campbell D. M. and Gillmer M. D. G. (1983) *Nutrition in Pregnancy*. London, Royal College of Obstetricians and Gynaecologists

Chamberlain G. (1980) The prepregnancy clinic. *Br. Med. J.* **281**, 29–30

Harley J. M. G. (Ed.) (1982) *Clinics in Obstetrics and Gynaecology: Preconception Clinics*. London, W. B. Saunders

Hawkins D. F. and Elder M. G. (1979) *Human Fertility Control*. London, Butterworths

Kohner N. (1984) *Pregnancy Book*. London, Health Education Council

Leading Article (1981) Preconception clinics. *Br. Med. J.* **283**, 685

Ledward R. S. and Hawkins D. F. (1983) *Drugs in Obstetrics*. London, Chapman & Hall

Pratt O. E. (Ed.) Mechanisms of alcohol damage in utero. Ciba Foundation Symposium, 105. London, Ciba Foundation

Rodec¹. C. H. and Nicolaides K. H. (Eds) (1984) *Prenatal Diagnosis*. London, Wiley & Sons

Smithell R. W., Sheppard S., Schorah C. *et al.* (1980) Possible prevention of neural tube defects by periconceptional vitamin supplement. *Lancet,* **i**, 339–340

Stewart Truswell A. (1983) Nutrition for pregnancy. *Br. Med. J.* **291**, 263–265

Chapter 2

Associated Medical and Surgical Disorders

INTRODUCTION

The ideal outcome of pregnancy is a healthy mother and healthy baby. When pregnancy is complicated by medical or surgical disease in the mother, it is necessary for the obstetrician to have an understanding of the relevant disease and, at the same time, to be able to liaise with the appropriate colleague.

This subject cannot be discussed in depth in this practical handbook and further reading is encouraged when specific problems arise, but common medical disorders that arise include pregnancy-induced hypertension (p. 60), diabetes mellitus and thyrotoxicosis, whilst in gynaecological practice sexually transmitted disease (p. 125), deep venous thrombosis (p. 157) and other disorders should be remembered.

DIABETES MELLITUS

The perinatal mortality in diabetic pregnancy can be two or three times that in non-diabetic pregnancy. Strict antenatal care, intrapartum fetal monitoring and intensive neonatal care help reduce the perinatal mortality rate and now pre-natal counselling (p. 6) is recommended for the established diabetic patient and routine screening tests at 28 weeks' gestation will help detect early onset of pregnancy-associated diabetes.

9

1. Glycosylated haemoglobin (HbA$_1$). Raised levels of HbA$_1$ in the first trimester may be associated with a raised incidence of congenital abnormality indicating specialized ultrasound screening.
2. Random blood glucose concentration (*see* Lindt and Anderson, 1984). A random blood glucose concentration is taken in the first antenatal clinic visit and also between 28 and 32 weeks' gestation. Blood levels in excess of 6·1 mmol/l within 2 hours after a meal or 5·6 mmol/l more than 2 hours after a meal indicate the need for a formal 75 g oral glucose tolerance test.
3. One hour blood glucose values. An alternative procedure is that all patients attend the antenatal clinic at 32 weeks gestation having had their normal breakfast. In the clinic 50 g of glucose is taken orally and after one hour a blood sugar result is taken together with blood for other appropriate investigations. During the one-hour delay, the patient can be assessed in the clinic. Blood sugar values above 6·1 mmol/l indicate the need for a formal 75 g glucose tolerance test.
4. Criteria for routine full glucose tolerance test include:
    a. Potential diabetic with past history of previous baby weighing more than 9 lbs.
    b. Obesity: more than 12% above ideal weight for height (*see Table* 1.1).
    c. Glycosuria on two or more occasions.
    d. Previous congenital abnormality, unexplained stillbirth or neonatal death.
    e. Hydramnios.
    f. Previous gestational diabetes.
    g. Positive family history.
    Referral to a combined diabetic/antenatal clinic supervised by consultant obstetrician and consultant physician specializing in diabetes mellitus is then indicated.

The presence of diabetes mellitus in pregnancy is associated with maternal fetal and neonatal complications including:

Maternal complications
   Infertility and spontaneous abortion.
   Pregnancy-induced hypertension.
   Hydramnios.
   Pre-term labour.

Fetal complications
   Increased perinatal mortality.
   Unexplained intra-uterine death.
   Congenital abnormality.

Neonatal complications
   Hypoglycaemia.
   Respiratory distress syndrome.
   Neonatal hypocalcaemia.
   Hyperbilirubinaemia.
   Renal vein thrombosis.
   Polycythaemia.

Hospital delivery in an obstetric and paediatric unit fully equipped to manage the pregnant diabetic patient is therefore essential.

OTHER ENDOCRINE DISORDERS

Pregnancy is not unknown in patients with other endocrine disorders, including hyperprolactinaemia from prolactinomas, diabetes insipidus, thyroid dysfunction, hyperparathyroidism or hypoparathyroidism. Many medical disorders are diagnosed prior to conception but all obstetricians should be alert to the possibility of endocrine abnormality. Below is given the management required for the different endocrine disorders.

Pituitary

Prolactinoma

Bromocriptine is indicated prior to conception and stopped when pregnancy is diagnosed. Visual field checks required every six weeks.

Hypopituitarism

Conventional hormone replacement therapy is continued during pregnancy.

Posterior Pituitary Disease

There may be deterioration in the diabetes insipidus with an increased requirement for extra desmopressin.

Thyroid

Hypothyroidism

Most patients receive 150–200 μg of L-thyroxine per day; thyroid function test should be reassessed prior to conception and at booking, 32 weeks and postnatal clinic.

Hyperthyroidism

This may first present during pregnancy and thyroid function tests (p. 163) are indicated on clinical suspicion (persistent tachycardia, weight loss, bruit in a goitre, exophthalmos, pretibial myxoedema). Abortion, pre-term labour and neonatal thyrotoxicosis may arise due to the transplacental passage of thyroid-stimulating immunoglobins.

Medical treatment using carbimazole or propylthiouracil is indicated in the first instance, and thyroidectomy if there is no improvement. Sympathomimetic drugs are contra-indicated and, if deterioration occurs during labour and the hyperthyroidism becomes severe, propanolol and iodide may be used.

Transient hypothyroidism may occur in the neonate. Neonatal thyrotoxicosis may also occur. Cord blood levels of T_4, free thyroxine concentration and T_3 should be determined. The mother's thyroid function should be monitored at day 8, postnatal clinic and at 4 months postpartum.

Adrenal Gland

Adrenal Cortical Hypofunction

The patients are maintained on 25–50 mg of hydrocortisone per day. An adrenal crisis may occur when nausea and vomiting may be mistaken for an early pregnancy.

Blood pressure, weight, blood urea, electrolytes and glucose concentration should be monitored at every ante-natal clinic visit. Parenteral hydrocortisone (200 mg i.m. or 100 mg i.v.) should be given every 6 hours throughout labour and reduced in the immediate postnatal period.

Breast feeding or oral contraception is not contra-indicated.

Adrenal Cortical Hyperfunction

There is a very high rate of fetal loss; the mother's health may be seriously jeopardized. Diagnosis is difficult due to pregnancy-associated changes in circulating cortisol and ACTH so computerized tomographic imaging of the adrenals and pituitary is indicated. Termination of pregnancy is indicated in the first trimester followed by definitive treatment. Treatment in the second trimester is either medical using metyrapone, or surgical.

Adrenal Medulla (Phaeochromocytoma)

This is a catecholamine-secreting tumour which can present as epileptiform fits, pregnancy-induced hypertension (p. 60) or abruptio placentae (p. 64). There is an increase in plasma or urinary catecholamines (adrenaline, nor-adrenaline, vanillyl mandelic acid).

Parathyroid Gland

Hyperparathyroidism

Treatment is indicated since there is a 50% pregnancy loss through abortion, intra-uterine death, pre-term delivery and neonatal tetany in untreated patients.

Treatment may be medical with oral phosphates or surgery during the second trimester. The neonate should be assessed for hypocalcaemia.

Hypoparathyroidism

The vitamin D analogue dihydrotachysterol 250–1000 mg per day, with 1–2 g of elemental calcium per day provides good prognosis. Serum calcium levels should be monitored at each antenatal clinic visit.

A hypocalcaemic crisis (severe tetany, pharyngeal spasm, fits), should be treated with a slow intravenous injection of calcium (10–20 ml of 10% calcium gluconate given at a rate of 10 ml/min and then by constant infusion, 10 ml of 10% calcium gluconate in 500 ml of Hartman's solution every 6 hours).

Breast feeding is contraindicated since vitamin D may cause infant hypervitaminosis.

CARDIOVASCULAR DISORDERS

Evidence of organic heart disease has been shown to exist in 0·4–4·1% of pregnant patients. Rheumatic heart disease is now rare in the UK, but congenital cardiac disease, cardiomyopathy and ischaemic heart disease may be evident. The haemodynamic effects of pregnancy with the associated increased cardiac output enables haemic cardiac murmurs to be diagnosed at an early stage in pregnancy and referral for probable further definitive diagnosis and advice regarding management is necessary.

Rheumatic heart disease will require antibiotic cover during surgical procedures (dental extraction or dental

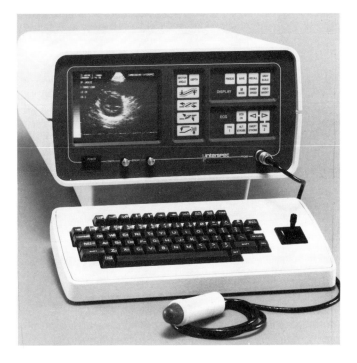

Fig. 2.1 Cardioscan high resolution cardiac sector scanner.

toilet, surgical induction of labour) and broad spectrum penicillin is indicated with gentamicin or streptomycin. Other cardiac drugs used during pregnancy include diuretics, digitalis, β-adrenergic receptor-blocking agents, anti-arrhythmic agents and α-adrenergic receptor stimulants. Delivery should be within hospital, with a spontaneous vaginal delivery being the preferred method. Lumbar epidural anaesthesia with outlet forceps delivery is advisable.

No surgical procedure, e.g. sterilization (p. 106) should be considered for approximately 3 months postpartum.

SURGICAL DISORDERS IN PREGNANCY

These present considerable difficulty in diagnosis because of altered anatomy and physiology and also in management because of potential risks of treatment (*see* Simmons and Luck, 1971).

Surgical disorders in pregnancy are fortunately rare, but should always be considered a differential diagnosis. The subject is extensive and further reading is mandatory but common problems that may confront the resident include those shown below.

Abdominal Pain

'. . . the commonest cause of abdominal pain in the pregnant patient is labour . . .'

Other diagnoses to be considered include abortion, abnormal placenta, pregnancy-induced hypertension and pre-eclampsia, degenerating leiofibromata, ovarian cysts undergoing torsion, acute appendicitis, intestinal obstruction, cholecystitis, nephrolithiasis, constipation.

Breast Lumps

These may be diagnosed during pregnancy necessitating surgical biopsy.

Pelvic Disorders

Ovarian cysts may require surgery for haemorrhage or twisting and surgery is best deferred until the second trimester.

Carcinoma of the Cervix

This may be diagnosed during pregnancy and a cervical smear is indicated at the booking clinic. A persistent vaginal discharge may not be benign and speculum examination of the cervix is essential.

Leiofibromata (fibroids)

These may complicate pregnancy by degeneration or obstruction in labour. Myomectomy is contraindicated during pregnancy.

SUMMARY

Where an associated medical or surgical disorder exists in addition to pregnancy, a combined medical–surgical–obstetric team is mandatory for good management.

FURTHER READING

Brudenell M. and Wilds P. L. (1984) *Medical and Surgical Problems in Obstetrics*. Bristol, Wrights

deSwiet M. (Ed.) (1984) *Medical Disorders in Obstetric Practice*. Oxford, Blackwell Scientific

deSwiet M. (1985) Some rare medical complications of pregnancy (leading article) *Br. Med. J.* **290**, 2–3

Lind T. and Anderson J. (1984) Does random blood glucose sampling outdate testing for glycosuria in the detection of diabetes during pregnancy. *Br. Med. J.* **289**, 1569

Simmons S. C. and Luck R. J. (Eds) (1971) *General Surgery in Gynaecological Practice.* Oxford, Blackwell Scientific

Chapter 3

Antenatal Clinics

INTRODUCTION

Antenatal clinics were widely established in the UK in 1918 and have been shown to play a significant role in the reduction of perinatal mortality. Whilst pre-pregnancy clinics may not be considered, as yet, to be of value by many women, antenatal clinics are more established and acceptable to most women in our community. In less sophisticated cultures, progress still has to be made in educating women to attend their doctor early and at regular intervals throughout their pregnancy. Improvements still need to be made within the National Health Service as regards the design of clinics, appointment systems and to resolving patients' main complaints of being attended to by different doctors and the lack of time for discussion. Each and every clinic must make self-assessment, and to reduce clinic congestion patients could be seen by their own general practitioners in association with hospital appointments ('shared care').

APPOINTMENTS

For healthy patients one suggested format for appointments is:
1. Hospital booking clinic: before 12 weeks (*see* p. 23).
2. First follow-up clinic at hospital at 16 weeks (*see* p. 26).
3. Further follow-up clinics at the general practitioner every 4 weeks until the next hospital visit at 32 weeks.

Further follow-up visits are as follows:

20 weeks—general practitioner
Clinical assessment
Haemoglobin
Weight
Urinalysis
Blood pressure

24 weeks—general practitioner
Clinical assessment
Haemoglobin
Weight
Urinalysis
Blood pressure

28 weeks—general practitioner
Clinical assessment
Haemoglobin
Weight
Urinalysis
Blood pressure
A certificate of confinement will be given

30 weeks—general practitioner
Clinical assessment
Haemoglobin
Weight
Urinalaysis
Blood pressure

4. Hospital visit at 32 weeks for a glucose screening test (after a standard diet, 50 g of glucose is taken and 2 hours later a blood sugar value recorded); if the 2 hours blood sugar is above 6.1 mmol/l the clinic midwife will contact the patient to reattend for a formal glucose tolerance test (p. 163). A fetal kick chart should be provided (Chapter 5).

5. Further follow-up clinic visits at the general practitioner every 2 weeks from 32 to 36 weeks.

6. Weekly visits to general practitioner until 39 weeks for the next *hospital assessment.*
7. Then a review by the *general practitioner* at 40 weeks.
8. Final *hospital visit* at term + 10 days for assessment regarding induction and delivery (*see* p. 60). (The expected date of delivery will be calculated from the initial ultrasound assessment.)

'SHARED CARE' PROTOCOLS

There will be many variations on this formula but it does allow a shared care programme with the general practitioner whilst specific hospital tests may still be monitored during the hospital visits. Such hospital visits will be increased where indicated and especially for those patients who may be designated as 'high risk pregnancies' (*see Table* 3.1) (Arias, 1984).

At all times, should a complication arise, the general practitioner could refer the patient to the next hospital antenatal clinic for reassessment.

Table 3.1. 'High-risk pregnancies'

Age under 20 years or over 35 years
Parity 4 or over
Multiple pregnancy
Previous history of premature birth or abortion
Previous history of stillbirth or neonatal death
Social class 5 or unsupported patients
Cigarette smokers, alcoholics, drug addicts
Renal disease
Hypertension, diabetes, medical disorders
Small for dates
Weight loss
History of infertility
'Sixth sense' by clinician

Patients in the 'high-risk' group will require serial placental function tests including fetal kick charts, serum oestriol, serum human placental lactogen, serial ultra-sonography to assess fetal growth by measuring the biparietal diameter (*see Fig.* 3.1) and cardiotokography (*see* Chapter 5).

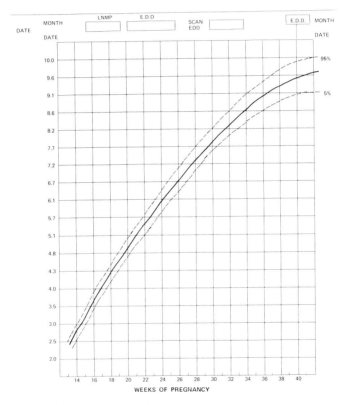

Fig. 3.1. Graph of biparietal diameters (in centimetres) during pregnancy.

Summary

The 'shared care' protocol ensures minimal visits to the hospital clinics. The patient can thus be supervised on a 1:1 basis by her own general practitioner and extra time is allowed for consultant supervision of the more complicated cases during the hospital visits (normally 3 or 4 visits). Crowding of antenatal clinics is thus minimized and unnecessary hospital visits (especially in rural areas) reduced. Antenatal clinic design faults should be reviewed.

Booking Clinics

These clinics are essential for:

1. Appropriate booking arrangements.
2. Confirmation of pregnancy—if necessary by ultra-sound.
3. Routine medical assessment of weight, height, general examination.
4. Initial investigations may include:

    Haemoglobin

    Blood group (patients should receive an inter-national blood group card)

    Serological tests for syphilis

    Rubella assessment (patients should receive a rubella assessment card)

    Antibody status

    Australian antigen for patients with a past history of hepatitis

    Haemoglobin electrophoresis

    Sickle-cell test

    Stool samples for oocytes

    Chest radiography if active tuberculosis is suspected

    Mid-stream specimen of urine

    Chorion villus biopsy between 8–12 weeks for chromosome analysis and enzyme studies on the fetus (Lui, 1986) (*see Fig.* 3.2).

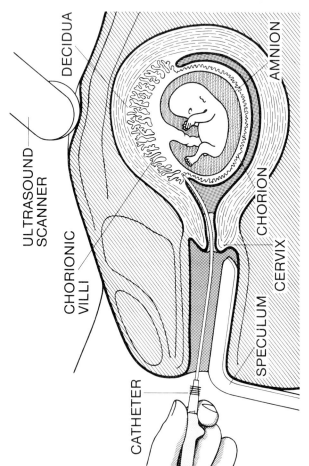

Fig. 3.2. Chorionic villus sampling catheter.

5. Exclusion of pelvic pathology involving vaginal assessment:
   Cervical swab
   Cervical smear.
6. Initial apprehensions may be allayed, questions answered, appropriate pregnancy care information booklets provided and advice given regarding diet, exercise, cigarettes, alcohol and drugs in pregnancy.

   A discussion on screening tests available for the exclusion of genetic abnormalities should be offered with reference to α-fetoprotein studies, ultrasonography, chorionic villus biopsy or amniocentesis (*Table* 3.2).

Table 3.2. Maternal age risk factors by one year intervals for Down's syndrome births

Maternal age (years)	Incidence
33	1/592
34	1/465
35	1/365
36	1/287
37	1/225
38	1/177
39	1/139
40	1/109
41	1/85
42	1/67
43	1/53
44	1/41
45	1/32
46	1/25
47	1/20
48	1/16
49	1/16
50	1/12

7. If any medical or surgical condition is discovered, referral to the appropriate specialist is mandatory, e.g. diabetes mellitus, thyrotoxicosis, congenital cardiac disease (*see* Chapter 2).

8. Contraception, whether this has been used in the past and any plans for the future, should be discussed during the antenatal clinics.

9. Obstetric analgesic procedures should be discussed (p. 80).

10. Mothercraft and parentcraft classes are available and patients and their husbands should be encouraged to attend; advice on when to discontinue work should be given.

11. Hospital or home delivery; the booking clinic will provide a manifest opportunity for stressing the advantages of hospital delivery.

Some patients now present their own 'birthplan' (*see Table* 3.3); they should be encouraged to visit the antenatal and postnatal wards, the labour ward and to attend parentcraft clinics, but if they decline hospital review the minimum that should be required is:

a. Initial booking clinic appointment.

b. Hospital delivery agreeing to all their wishes including a 6-hour discharge.

First Follow-up Hospital Visit at 16 weeks

1. A review of the results available should be made.

2. The patients' questions and apprehensions should be discussed.

3. Blood should be taken for an α-fetoprotein assessment.

4. A pelvic ultrasound examination should be undertaken and repeated two or three times routinely during the pregnancy at approximately 32 and 39 weeks for serial growth, placentography and presentation of the fetus.

Table 3.3. 'Birthplan'

Name:

Antenatal classes:

	Would like:	*Wish to avoid:*
On admission	Own nightdress	Enema Shave Induction (unless medically necessary)

During labour	Partner present *at all times*
	Use of 'birth room'
	  (if available)
	Bath/shower
	Mobility
	Music (will provide own tapes)
	Rocking chair (if available)?
		Artificial rupture of
		  membranes
		Continuous electronic
		  monitoring
		Intravenous drip

Pain killers	Gas and air, if requested	Pethidine ⎫ But, if decided upon, Epidural ⎬ timed to wear off ⎭ before delivery

Delivery	Partner to be present,
	  at all times
	Upright position
	  (will bring own 'birth stool')
	Gentle pushing (have practised)
	Dim room
	Lift baby out by self
	Baby delivered onto abdomen
	Cord cut when stopped pulsing
	Baby bath ready
	Time for us to spend with baby
		Episiotomy
		Lying flat on back
		Deliberate breath holding

In case of caesarean	Epidural, if available, with partner present and baby delivered to breast	'Automatic' caesarean for a breech baby Only if absolutely necessary
Feeding	Breast feeding Feeding on demand	To be separated from baby (unless exhausted and in need of sleep!) 'Top-ups' or glucose

To date, no studies have confirmed any deleterious effects from diagnostic ultrasound to the fetus or mother.

Hospital delivery remains the only safe situation to deliver a baby and all mothers should be encouraged to accept hospital delivery involving, where necessary, domino delivery, general practitioner units, birthing room facilities.

MEDICAL SOCIAL WORKER

Potentially the maternity department offers one of the best opportunities for preventive social work in the community and a positive contribution to the well-being of the family. The birth of a baby constitutes a life crisis and, according to crisis theory, the individual is most susceptible to change in crisis. Modern research confirms that stress during pregnancy, and particularly marital stress, is associated with a very much higher rate of physical handicap and emotional maladjustment in the offspring. Further, certain factors have been demonstrated to be significant in child abuse situations. Children of very young mothers, the premature, sick or otherwise damaged children, especially those who have been cared for in the special care baby unit, seem to be especially vulnerable.

The social work department offers counselling and help and advice throughout the pregnancy and afterwards, if necessary. The social worker will offer termination counselling and follow-up; also advice on possible adoption and fostering. He/she may offer help and advice with environmental and financial problems and will liaise with the appropriate central/local government or voluntary services, where necessary. The social worker will also discuss any anxieties or worries which may be troubling the mother and her family. Almost certainly, good care and support of the mother during her pregnancy will help her to establish positive feelings towards her offspring.

Mothers whose babies are in the special care unit very often have other responsibilities at home and leave hospital after a few days. The high cost of public transport may inhibit frequent visiting and the social worker may help in this matter by liaising with the Department of Health and Social Security, where possible, and otherwise by making applications for grants to various voluntary bodies.

Sometimes a sick mother may require home help support for a while following delivery and, in certain cases, the Family Welfare Service is available for mothers who experience difficulty in household management and child care. Parents of handicapped babies sometimes require on-going support and counselling. Similarly, those couples whose babies were stillborn may be appropriately referred to give them the opportunity to talk about their loss.

AMNIOCENTESIS

An amniocentesis, if required, will be undertaken at 16 weeks. Normally an outpatient procedure, this should be performed under aseptic conditions with ultrasound control. Full counselling, including an explanation of the risk to the fetus, is important.

Procedure

Local anaesthesia (10 ml of 1% lignocaine) is used and a 20 gauge spinal needle used. The tap should be clear. The patient is asked to rest for half an hour afterwards.

Indications

In the First Trimester
1. For karyotyping in cases at risk of Down's syndrome (aged 35 or over, *see Table* 3.2) or other chromosomal

abnormality, especially where either partner is known to carry any form of chromosome translocation.

2. Some hereditary metabolic disorders.

3. Raised maternal serum α-fetoprotein (MSAP), to detect neural tube defect [associated with raised liquor α-fetoprotein and abnormal acetyl cholinesterase (ACh band)].

4. For presence of glia or neuronal cells—indicative of an open neural tube defect.

In Mid Trimester and Third Trimester

In cases of rhesus disease, it is performed to detect a rising antibody titre, and to determine a raised lecithin–sphingo-myelin ratio (for fetal lung maturity) prior to delivery.

PROPHYLACTIC IRON AND FOLIC ACID THERAPY

To debate the place and need for prophylactic iron and folic acid therapy *see* Ledward and Hawkins (1983).

FURTHER READING

Arias F. (Ed.) (1984) *High Risk Pregnancy and Delivery.* St Louis, Miss., Mosby

Campbell S. (1969) The prediction of fetal maturity by ultrasonic measurement of the biparietal diameter. *J. Obstet. Gynaecol. Br. Commonw.* **76**, 603–609

Gordon Y. B. (Ed.) (1977) Clinical applications of immunoassay to pregnancy. *J. Mat. Child. Hlth,* **2** (6), 218

Leading Article (1977) Diagnostic amniocentesis in early pregnancy. *Br. Med. J.* **1**, 1430–1431

Ledward R. S. and Hawkins D. F. (1983) *Drug Treatment in Obstetrics.* London, Chapman & Hall

Lui D. Y., Golbus M. S. and Symonds E. M. (1986) *Chorionic Villus Biopsy.* London, Chapman & Hall

Chapter 4

Antenatal Wards

INTRODUCTION

An opportunity to visit the antenatal wards will be provided when the patient attends the booking clinic, antenatal clinic or normally the parentcraft classes. Such opportunities allow parents to meet the antenatal ward staff and hopefully (normally in 85% of patients), no further visit will be required. However, admission to the antenatal wards may be required and explanation of the reason for admission is a major part of therapy. Admission to hospital should be a last resort where observation and treatment is not suitable at home, especially where the family unit may be disturbed for several weeks.

ADMISSION TO HOSPITAL: INDICATIONS AND MANAGEMENT

The following are examples for admission to the antenatal ward and the Resident should clerk the patient and commit himself to a diagnosis and appropriate management plan informing the Registrar where indicated:

Indications	*Management*
1. Patients who are 'small for dates'	Bed rest and placental function tests, daily cardiotokography (Chiswick, 1985)

2. Pregnancy induced hyper-tension, renal disease (p. 60)

Bed rest, mild sedation, consider hypotensive drugs, placental and renal function tests, daily cardiotokography

3. Anaemia (patients with persistent low haemoglobin level of < 10 g/dl)

Moderate ambulation, investigate haemoglobin, blood film, serum iron, folate, serum vitamin B_{12}; Hb electrophoresis; stool for oocyte; mid-stream specimen of urine
Discuss with haematologist
Consider sternal marrow and need for total dose iron infusion

4. Oligohydramnios Polyhydramnios

Bed rest, placental function tests, daily cardiotokography

5. Antepartum haemorrhage (p. 64)

Bed rest, placental function tests, daily cardiotokography
Placental location by ultrasound; group 2 units of blood and hold in reserve

6. Medical problems associated with pregnancy; cardiac disease, thyroid disorders, diabetes mellitus (Chapter 2)

Management in consultation with medical colleagues

7. Multiple pregnancy (Weekes et al., 1977)

Admission is *not* routinely indicated at 28–32 weeks; hospital admission is normally indicated where there is a clinical suspicion of pre-term labour or where maternal distress exists
Bed rest, monitor haemoglobin and serum for folate levels
Placental function tests using serial

	ultrasonography, consider induction after 38 weeks' gestation
8. Abnormal lie of fetus	Bed rest, placentography using ultrasound, consider elective caesarean section after 38 weeks' gestation
9. Rhesus negative with antibodies	Consider transfer to regional centre for appropriate investigations
10. Premature rupture of membranes (p. 70)	*a.* Bed rest in hospital
	b. Observe for confirmation of ruptured membranes (pyridium/ methylene blue tests)
	c. Observe for early pre-term labour (*see* p. 58)
	d. Consider antibiotic therapy only if there is clinical or bacterio- logical evidence of infection This may indicate fetal abnormality and ultrasonic scanning and/or abdominal radiographs are advised Should patients (between 24–36 weeks) with premature rupture of membranes go into labour, they should be transferred to the Regional Obstetric/Neonatal Unit Any vaginal interference should be at the direction of the consultant concerned All cases should wear a pad all the time to monitor loss Corticosteroids to stimulate surfactant may be considered (Ledward and Hawkins, 1983)

> *e.* Deliver at 34 weeks' gestation if there is persistent evidence of infection
>
> *f.* Consider classical incision if caesarean section is required.

Summary

The RMO should fully inform the patient and her husband as to the indication for the patient's admission and discuss fully the management of her case.

FURTHER READING

Chiswick M. L. (1985) Intrauterine growth retardation. *Br. Med. J.* **291**, 845–847

Ledward R. S. and Hawkins D. F. (1983) *Drug Treatment in Obstetrics*, p. 117 London, Chapman & Hall

Weekes A. R. L., Menzies D. N. and De Boer C. H. (1977) The relative efficacy of bed rest, cervical suture and no treatment in the management of twin pregnancy. *Br. J. Obstet. Gynaecol.* **84**, 161–164

Chapter 5

Fetal Monitoring

INTRODUCTION

All patients should be offered fetal monitoring, especially those patients in the 'high risk' category (*Table* 3.1). Methods of placental function tests include the following.

ANTENATAL

Clinical Assessment

Serial assessment of uterine growth should be monitored.

Fetal Kick Chart

The clinical value of a 12-hour daily fetal movement count has been shown to be of value in detecting early fetal asphyxia (Pearson and Weaver, 1976). Where the fetal kick frequency is reduced review and cardiotokography is indicated (*see Fig*. 5.1).

Serial Oestriol Values

This is a test of placental function (*see Fig*. 5.2 and *Table* 5.1). Isolated values are of little value but serial values are of use for defined high risk conditions such as diabetes, intra-uterine growth retardation or hypertension.

Drugs, ampicillin, hexamine, corticosteroids, may affect the results. This test can be performed on (*a*) a 24 hour collection of urine (*see Table* 5.1) or (*b*) a maternal blood sample.

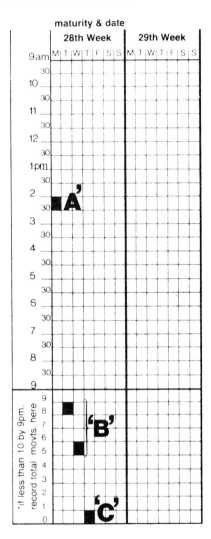

Fig. 5.1. The Cardiff 'count-to-ten' fetal activity chart.

Table 5.1. SI values for pregnancy oestrogens (urinary values)

Gestation (weeks)	Expected levels μmol/24 h	Borderline levels
30	24–92	12–23
31	24–95	12–23
32	30–101	16–29
33	33–109	16–32
34	38–121	21–37
35	43–135	21–42
36	47–158	24–46
37	52–164	29–51
38	56–201	35–55
39	61–215	38–60
40	69–226	47–68

Serum values may also be used.

Serial Human Placental Lactogen (HPL) Values

This too is a test of placental function (*see Table* 5.2, *Fig.* 5.3). HPL is synthesized and stored in the syncytio-trophoblast cell of the placenta.

Fetal Cardiotokography

Antenatal cardiotokography (*see Figs.* 5.4–5.6) has superseded serial oestriol and HPL levels in many centres. In other centres it is kept in reserve for patients with low placental function tests or impaired fetal kick charts when hospital admission and serial cardiotokography is undertaken.

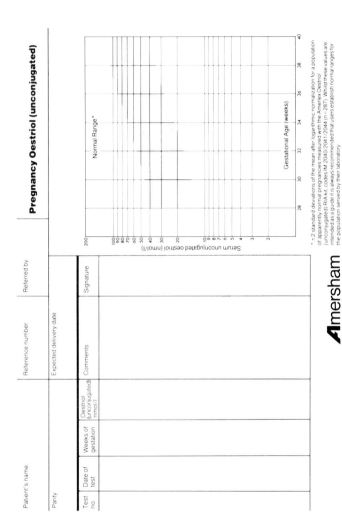

Fig. 5.2. Chart for serial oestrogen values.

Table 5.2. Human placental lactogen levels

Weeks of pregnancy	No. of samples	Mean (µg/ml)	s.d.	2 × s.d.
22	37	2·1	0·4	0·8
24	41	2·7	0·5	1·0
26	49	2·9	0·5	1·0
28	26	3·6	0·7	1·4
30	27	4·1	0·5	1·0
32	23	4·4	0·6	1·2
34	22	4·9	0·5	1·0
36	12	5·5	0·6	1·2
37	23	5·7	0·7	1·4
38	33	5·5	1·0	2·0
39	29	5·3	1·0	2·0
40	32	5·5	1·0	2·0
41	19	5·2	0·7	1·4
42	11	4·7	0·7	1·4

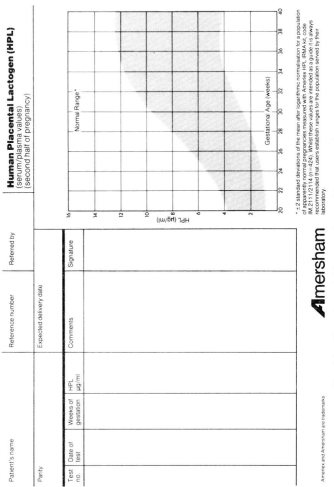

Fig. 5.3. Chart for serial human placental lactogen values.

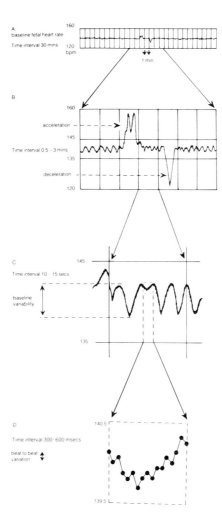

Fig. 5.4. Four orders of fetal heart rate variation.

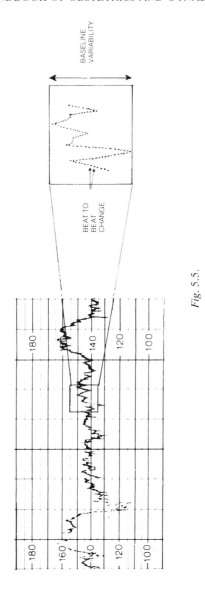

Fig. 5.5.

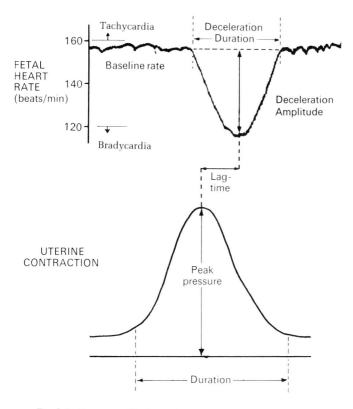

Fig. 5.6. Terms used in the study of continuous records of FHR.

INTRAPARTUM

Not all patients will accept fetal monitoring, especially since it involves reduced mobility. Mobile fetal assessment equipment is less than satisfactory. All patients should, however, be offered fetal monitoring, including:

1. Clinical assessment.
2. Cardiotokography.
3. Fetal blood sampling (*see below*).

Cardiotokography

Definitions

Four orders of description of the continuous fetal heart rate (FHR) trace can be made (*Fig.* 5.4).

a. Even intermittent or imperfect sampling of the FHR will allow the construction of an average baseline rate. This has been done for many years using the Pinard stethoscope.

b. Fluctuations of the FHR from the baseline, greater than 15 beats/min are called 'accelerations' (increase in rate) or 'decelerations' (decrease in rate).

c. Regular fluctuations in baseline rate occur, usually with an amplitude of less than 15 beats/min (normal range 5–15 beats/min), and with between 3 and 5 complete cycles/min. This is called baseline variability. Each fluctuation contains between 25 and 40 individual beats, and has frequently been *incorrectly* called 'beat-to-beat' variation.

d. Beat-to-beat changes are usually less than 1 beat/min in amplitude, and cannot normally be seen on the CTG tracing, unless the change of rate is rapid and the tracing of superlative quality (*Fig.* 5.5). The clinical value of beat-to-beat heart rate variation measurement is not yet fully established.

Baseline F/H Rate

Normal baseline rate is from 120 to 160 beats/min. Rates from 100 to 120 beats/min can be considered normal if no other abnormalities are present.

1. Tachycardia: a heart rate with a baseline in excess of 160 beats/min is referred to as a tachycardia.
2. Bradycardia: if the baseline is less than 120 beats/min, it is called a bradycardia.

Accelerations

Increases in rate of more than 15 beats/min. Usually associated with fetal movement. In general, a reassuring sign indicating a healthy fetus.

Decelerations

Decreases in rate of more than 15 beats/min (*Fig*. 5.6). They are of two main types:

a. Reflex decelerations synchronous with uterine contractions.
b. Decelerations due to hypoxia, which are characterized by a 'lag time' in which the nadir (lowest point) of the deceleration is delayed with respect to the peak of the contraction. They are usually called 'late decelerations', once the lag time exceeds 15 seconds.

Fetal Blood Sampling

Fetal blood sampling is a technique which is used for obtaining capillary blood from the presenting part of the fetus during labour (*see Fig*. 5.8 for equipment used).

Clinical Indications for Collection of a Fetal Blood Sample

Clinical fetal distress is when:

1. Fetal heart rate more than 160 beats/min or less than 120 beats/min.

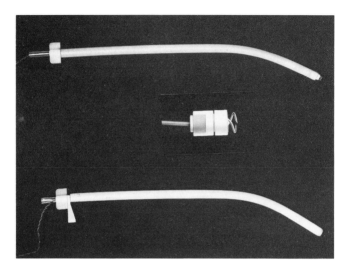

Fig. 5.7.   Fetal scalp electrodes for fetal monitoring.

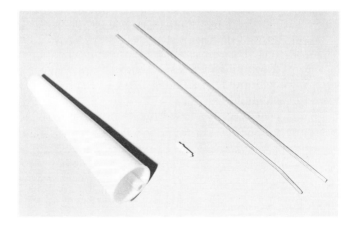

Fig. 5.8.   Equipment for fetal blood samples.

2. Meconium-stained liquor—artificial rupture of membrane in early established labour should be performed, when feasible, in order to detect this important sign.
3. Abnormal FH traces on monitoring.

SERIAL COLLECTION OF FBS While the severity of acidosis, indicated by the actual pH, is probably the most important aid in the diagnosis of fetal asphyxia, the observation of *changes* in pH of fetal samples collected serially may be helpful. For this reason, the following indications for the collection of further fetal samples are proposed: *repeat immediately* if (*a*) fetal pH <7·255; or (*b*) if the FHR abnormality, other than severe bradycardia, persists.

Techniques

1. The sterile pack containing the equipment should be opened, the blade screwed into the holder, the silicone jelly placed on a swab and holder, and the heparinized glass tube attached to the rubber tubing. With the patient in the lithotomy position, unless this causes worsening fetal distress, a routine vaginal examination should be made to determine:

   a. Dilatation and position of the cervix.
   b. Level of the presenting part in relation to the ischial spines.
   c. The nature and position of the presenting part.

2. Following the vaginal examination, the appropriate size of endoscope is introduced into the vagina along the palm of the right hand and right forefinger into the cervical canal. When in position the obturator is removed and the lighting unit clipped on to the lip of the endoscope.

3. The left hand now controls the endoscope and lighting unit. The external end of the endoscope is depressed to

elevate the narrow end which should be at right angles to the presenting part (this prevents liquor or cervix from entering the operative field). The endoscope should be rested against the presenting part with the minimum of pressure to avoid producing venous congestion.

4. A note should be made of the colour of the fetal skin at this time. A 'pink' scalp suggests that the fetus is well oxygenated, although a pallid scalp is not necessarily associated with fetal asphyxia.

5. The presenting part is cleaned with a swab and then sprayed with ethyl chloride. Silicone jelly is then wiped onto the presenting part with a swab. At least 15 seconds should elapse between the ethyl chloride spray and incising the presenting part.

6. Fetal blood samples (FBS) should be collected. This is most easily done during a uterine contraction, but this is not essential.

7. To make the incision, rest the blade on the skin and then pierce the skin. Very little force is needed for this. A single incision is usually all that is required, but occasionally a further incision may be necessary. At the most two incisions, which are close together, should be made. The best site of incision is at about 12 o'clock.

8. (a) Suction into the glass tubing must be controlled and the tip of the tube must be in the globule of the capillary blood though not in contact with the skin. Failure to observe these precautions will result in a specimen fragmented with air. Prolonged exposure of the globule of blood to the air results in loss of CO_2. (b) Do not spend more than five minutes after the first incision trying to obtain blood. The acid–base values are of little use after this time. It is important to recognize that the more difficult it is to collect a FBS, the less likely are acid–base values derived from this sample to

be representative of the true condition of the fetus. For this reason, essential honesty is needed to decide on the values of each sample in the clinical management of fetal distress. If difficulty in FBS collection is encountered, a satisfactory FBS can often be obtained by someone more experienced in the technique.

9. After collecting the FBS, the bleeding point should be lightly compressed with a dry swab until haemostasis has been secured. In the second stage, it may be necessary to leave the swab on the scalp until after delivery.

10. It is essential for the sample to be well mixed with the aid of the metal rod and magnet as soon as possible after collection. Failure to do so may result in clot formation. A member of the nursing staff is usually able to do this for you.

11. Maternal cubital vein blood: anticoagulate a 2-ml syringe by filling with heparin and then emptying it. If possible, do not compress the arm in order to distend the vein, but if this is necessary it is essential to wait a few seconds after releasing the compression before withdrawing blood from the vein.

12. Results should be entered on to the partogram (p. 56).

MISCELLANEOUS

Research methods occasionally used include:

1. Fetal breathing movements.
2. Meconium staining of amniotic fluid.
3. Antepartum stress monitoring.
4. Alkaline phosphatase.
5. Cysteine aminopeptidase.
6. Oxytocinase.
7. α-Fetoprotein.
8. Ultrasound assessment of umbilical cord flow.

FURTHER READING

Beard R. W. (Ed.) (1974) *Fetal Medicine. Clinics in Obstetrics and Gynaecology.* **1**(1)

Beard R. W. (1974) *Fetal Heart Patterns and Their Clinical Interpretations.* Chichester, Sonicaid Ltd

Pearson J. F. and Weaver J. B. (1976) Fetal activity and fetal wellbeing: an evaluation. *Br. Med. J.* **1**, 1305–1307

Quilligan E. J. (1979) *Update on Fetal Monitoring. Clinics in Obstetrics and Gynaecology,* **6**(2)

Chapter 6

The Labour Ward

INTRODUCTION

With the increasing demands for home delivery, patients should be encouraged to visit the hospital labour ward to meet and discuss with staff midwives any particular apprehensions that either partner may have. Labour wards should be made less clinical with extra 'birthing room' facilities, extra colour for delivery rooms and extra pictures and paintings, whilst maintaining safety features.

Patients should preferably be allocated a single midwife throughout their labour and husbands allowed to participate in the first stage management.

Hospital delivery is encouraged.

ADMISSION OF PATIENTS TO THE LABOUR SUITE

The resident medical officer (RMO) on duty should aim to see every patient before delivery, preferably within half an hour of her being admitted. At night, this would be at the night sister's discretion. The RMO should see any case which falls into a special category (*see* p. 58) immediately on admission.

Each morning a working labour ward round should be taken by the registrar and duty resident and include medical students on take. Combined rounds with the anaesthetic and paediatric registrars are encouraged to supervise potential problem cases. When patients elect minimal medical involvement, a social introduction and clinical assessment is all that is required.

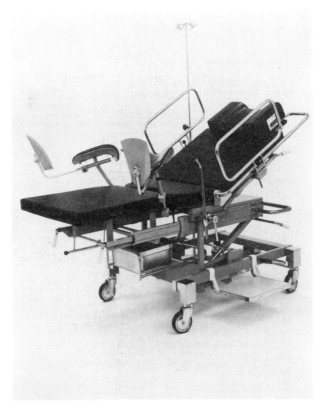

Fig. 6.1. Obstetric bed/chair.

MANAGEMENT OF NORMAL (OR CHOSEN/NATURAL) LABOUR

Definition

Patients with uncomplicated pregnancies who are in spontaneous labour between 38 and 42 weeks.

The management can differ in various units and 'normal' labour can be considered as 'natural' labour where there is a minimal involvement by the medical staff, or 'chosen' labour where the patient elects certain provisos (*see Table 3.3*, p. 27) after discussion of her management between herself and consultant obstetrician during the antenatal period.

First Stage

Vaginal examinations are obligatory on all patients (on admission to the labour suite) unless there is a contra-indication, for example:

1. APH.
2. Unstable lie and subsequently.
   a. On rupture of the membranes;
   b. at the midwife's discretion;
       i. when sedation or an epidural is required.
       ii. when it is thought that the patient is fully dilated.
   c. At least every four hours during active labour.
   d. Unexplained fetal distress.

The vaginal examinations may be undertaken by the midwife in charge or the RMO.

The membranes should be ruptured on the first vaginal examination when the head is engaged and the cervix is effaced and 3 cm or more dilated. An internal fetal scalp electrode for monitoring is advisable.

Analgesia (Moir, 1982)

a. Pethidine 100–150 mg ⎫ May be given by
  intramuscular injection
  Sparine 50 mg ⎬ and repeated after 3 hours
  or up to a maximum 2 doses
  Mepyramine 50 mg ⎭ before further review by
  (Phenergan) the RMO

Midwives are legally authorized to administer pethidine or pentazocine for analgesia but in hospital their action must be countersigned by a doctor within 12 h.

b. Continuous patient controlled infusions for analgesia should be considered.

c. Epidural analgesia (*see* p. 80).

Epidural analgesia may be offered to patients:
  i. In the antenatal clinic.
  ii. By the admitting RMO who should ensure appropriate explanation of the procedure is given.

Patients electing for epidural analgesia should give their informed verbal consent.

d. Some patients decline drugs for analgesia.

Diet

For patients in established labour, plain water only should be given. An intravenous 5% dextrose or Hartman's infusion may be considered.

Antacids

Magnesium trisilicate mixture 10 ml should be given every 2 hours and also preoperatively; alternatively 0·33 M citrate may be used. (*See also* p. 82).

Ranitid (Zantac) 10 mg i.m. dose for 12 hours is another alternative antacid.

Bath
A shower or ordinary bath may be given.

Shaving
No perineal shaving should be given.

Enemas
Patients should only have an enema if the rectum is loaded.

Supervision
Patients should never be left alone at any time in labour. Husbands are encouraged to remain in the labour ward throughout labour if they wish, but must understand that they will be expected to leave if requested to do so by a member of the nursing or medical staff.

Fetal Monitoring
All patients at risk should be monitored (p. 21).

Records
The pulse and fetal heart rate and uterine contractions are recorded every 30 minutes. The maternal blood pressure should be taken at least every hour. The urine must be tested for acetone and proteinuria at the time of voiding, when the patient is in labour. The presence of ketonuria should be treated by increasing the fluid intake using normal dextrose saline. All records should be charted on the partogram (*see* p. 56).

Oxytocin Stimulation
This should be considered if labour lies 2 hours to the right of the normal partogram chart (*Fig.* 6.2).

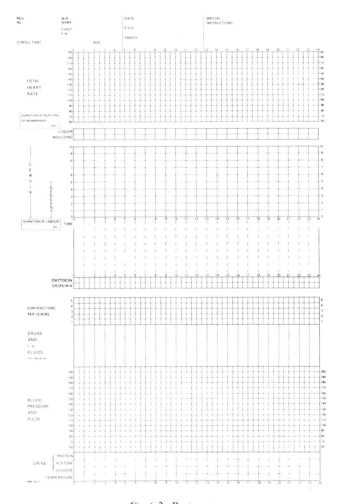

Fig. 6.2. Partogram.

Second Stage

Position

The dorsal position is the one most usually employed but some centres prefer the lateral, or even the squatting position.

Analgesia

Entonox (nitrous oxide, 50%; oxygen 50%) may be used routinely usually in the late first or in the second stage of labour in addition to the charted analgesia. If this is still insufficient, the RMO should be called to advise on further analgesia. (*See* Moir, 1982.)

Records

The blood pressure should be taken every 15 minutes; the maternal pulse and the fetal heart should be taken after every contraction if possible. If the patient is not on a monitor, the fetal heart should be checked every 5 minutes.

Length of Second Stage

Primigravida patients should usually be delivered within 1 hour and multigravida patients within 30 minutes. Medical aid is sought if there is any delay in progress.

Episiotomy

Mediolateral episiotomies (p. 99) are advised after 10 ml of local 1% lignocaine without adrenaline has been injected into the perineum. Medical students may undertake the episiorrhaphy after supervision by the RMO. Soluble sutures should be used for the episiorrhaphy.

Third Stage

Intramuscular Syntometrine (oxytocin + ergometrine) 1 ml or oxytocin (Syntocinon) 10 IU i.v. should be given by the midwife with the delivery of the anterior shoulder. Intravenous ergometrine is only given in an emergency or if specially ordered, e.g. in the case of a sudden postpartum haemorrhage or manual removal of placenta in patients whose haemoglobin is 10·0 g/dl or less. Oxytocin alone should be used for patients with hypertension or cardiac patients (Vaughan Williams *et al.*, 1974).

MANAGEMENT OF ABNORMALITIES ENCOUNTERED IN THE LABOUR WARD

The RMO should definitely see all patients in the categories below and discuss his management with the registrar—if for any reason the RMO is not obtained quickly, the midwife in charge should contact the registrar direct. All patients should have 2 units of blood cross matched on patient's admission in case emergency caesarean section is necessary.

Pre-term Labour (i.e. before 37 weeks)

Transfer in utero

Patients in pre-term labour between 24 and 36 weeks gestation and booked for a hospital delivery with limited neonatal resources may be transferred to the Regional Obstetric/Neonatal Unit after consultation with the consultant and obstetric registrar on duty at the regional centre.

Notes should accompany the patient to the regional centre with the request that they be returned at the earliest convenience.

Suppression of Uterine Activity

Many regimes are available to suppress labour:

i.   General sedation with pethidine (single dose).
ii. Ethanol.
iii. Prostaglandin synthetase inhibitors.
iv. Sympathomimetics, e.g. salbutamol or ritodrine.

SELECTION OF PATIENTS All patients presenting in spontaneous premature labour without evidence of amnionitis, thyrotoxicosis or cardiac disease should be selected. The physician should be satisfied that premature labour has commenced, i.e. regular contractions occurring at intervals of 10 minutes or less. Salbutamol treatment will then be started immediately.

ASSESSMENT BEFORE SALBUTAMOL TREATMENT Cervical dilatation or effacement will be recorded on the record form together with maternal blood pressure, pulse rate and fetal heart rate.

COMPOSITION OF SALBUTAMOL INFUSION An injection of 5 ml or 5 mg salbutamol should be added to 500 ml 5% dextrose solution to give a concentration of 10 μg salbutamol/ml, equivalent to 15 drops from a normal giving set.

ADMINISTRATION Patients will receive an infusion of salbutamol through a forearm vein. The infusion will be started at 10 drops/min (6·7 μg salbutamol/min) and increased by 10-drop increments at 5–10 min intervals until contractions cease or an infusion rate of 50 drops/min (33 μg/min) is reached. If contractions have not ceased, the infusion will be increased by 10-drop increments at 20-min intervals. Treatment should be stopped if any of the following occur:

i.   An infusion rate of 80 drops/min (53 μg/min

salbutamol) does not reduce contractions in strength, duration or frequency.

ii. The cervix has dilated significantly after six hours of treatment.

iii. A steady maternal pulse rate exceeding 140 per min is reached.

Once the contractions have ceased, the infusion will be maintained at this steady rate for one hour. The infusion rate will then be reduced by half and maintained at this lower rate for six hours. The infusion rate will then be reduced by half again and maintained for a further six hours before starting oral treatment with 4 mg salbutamol four times daily for one week.

SIDE-EFFECTS In the event of unacceptable side-effects occurring, such as tremor or palpitations, salbutamol dosage by infusion or oral routes may be reduced.

Prevention of Respiratory Distress Syndrome

Corticosteroids may be prescribed after discussion with the consultant.

'Small for Dates' fetus

Fetal monitoring is required.

Pregnancy-induced Hypertension

Pre-eclampsia

Patients are admitted to the antenatal ward for rest, placental function tests and normally surgical induction of labour when the fetus is mature at 37–38 weeks' gestation or if there is a deterioration in the hypertensive state or if albuminuria deteriorates.

During the antenatal period hypotensive therapy with methyldopa or labetalol is in vogue but, for intrapartum use, alternative managements available include (*see* Ledward and Hawkins, 1983; deSwiet, 1985):

i. Epidural analgesia.
ii. Diazepam.
iii. Apresoline.
iv. Lytic cocktails, e.g.
      Pethidine   = 50 mg ⎫
      Promethazine   = 50 mg ⎬ by injection
      Chlorpromazine = 50 mg ⎭
v. Chlormethiazole edisylate.
vi. Magnesium sulphate.

If magnesium sulphate is elected, the RMO should monitor the reflexes, respiratory rate and urinary output; 10% calcium gluconate should be available as an antidote.

The RMO should inform the registrar who will discuss the case with the consultant concerned.

Fulminating Pre-eclampsia

i.   Inform the registrar before starting treatment. A full general medical assessment of the patient should be undertaken to exclude coarctation of the aorta, renal artery stenosis, phaeochromocytoma (24 hour urine test for vanillyl mandelic acid) and renal disease (renal function tests).
ii.   Commence regular pulse and blood pressure readings.
iii. Continuous bladder drainage.
iv.   Strict fluid balance charts should be maintained.
v.   Monitor the patient and the fetus.
vi.   Mannitol 10% is the preferred diuretic for fluid retention.
vii. Consider delivery of fetus by vaginal delivery or caesarean section.

viii. Consider possibility of disseminated intravascular coagulopathy.
ix. Keep the consultant on duty informed.

Eclampsia

i. The consultant on duty must be kept informed.
ii. Diazepam 10 mg i.v. stat and 10 mg i.m. stat should be given.
iii. Maintain an open airway.
iv. Consider alternative diagnoses.

Anaemia (Haemoglobin less than 10 g/dl)

Fetal monitoring required. Group 2 units of blood in reserve.

Elderly Primigravida (over 30 years)

Fetal monitoring required. Consider epidural analgesia if available.

Very Young Primigravida (below 16 years)

Consider epidural analgesia if available.

Cases of Subfertility/Poor Obstetric History

Fetal monitoring required. Consider epidural analgesia if available.

All Patients with Previous Caesarean Section Scar or Previous Myomectomy/Hysterotomy Scar

Trial of labour where the caesarean section was performed for a non-recurring condition, e.g. placenta praevia. Where

oxytocin is indicated for multiparous patients who have had previous caesarean section. Fetal and maternal monitoring (p. 71). Monitor pulse rate. (Tachycardia may indicate rupture of the scar.)

All Abnormal Presentations or Unstable Lies
Discuss with registrar.

Multiple Pregnancies
Consider epidural analgesia.

Patients with Medical History
Fetal monitoring is required for those having a medical history of any of the following:
a. Cardiac disease.
b. Diabetes.
c. Any previous severe medical or surgical history.

Oligohydramnios, Polyhydramnios
Fetal monitoring is required.

Maternal or Fetal Condition

Ketosis in Labour
Correction by intravenous dextrose (5–10%) is required.

Maternal Distress
In maternal distress, i.e. tachycardia of 120, or clinical opinion—assess the progress of labour—consider fetal blood sampling.

Fetal Distress

i.   Fetal heart rate more than 160.
ii. Fetal heart rate less than 120.
iii. Irregular fetal heart rate; type I and type II deceler-
     ations; lack of beat-to-beat variation (*see* p. 44, *Table*
     5.4).
iv. Meconium—fresh or stale.

Fetal distress will indicate the need for cardiotokography, or possibly fetal blood sampling.

Intra-uterine Death

A coagulation disorder may arise with this problem but it
normally occurs some considerable time after the death of
the fetus and definitive evidence of death must be obtained
prior to evacuation of the uterus.

i.   No fetal heart audible.
ii. Failure of growth (BPD) on serial ultrasonic scanning.
iii. Radiographic evidence (Spalding's sign).

Blood should be taken weekly for coagulation factors
and when definite evidence of death is found the uterus
may be evacuated using prostaglandins (p. 135).

i. Psychotherapy for puerperal depression will be required.
ii. Bromocriptine should be considered to suppress
    lactation (p. 92).

Antepartum Haemorrhage, Intrapartum Haemorrhage

Fetal monitoring is required. Abruptio placentae (acci-
dental haemorrhage), placenta praevia or local causes, e.g.
vasa previa or a heavy 'show' should all be considered.

Resuscitation, if required, should be initiated and the
registrar informed. Any vaginal interference should be at

the direction of the consultant concerned. Routine investigations will include haemoglobin, packed cell volume, group and cross-match and coagulation factors requested if a coagulation failure is considered probable (discuss with the haematologists.

With a probable placenta praevia, placental localization will be required (*see* p. 187) when the bleeding has stopped.

All patients should wear a pad at the time to monitor loss.

An examination under anaesthesia in the operating room may be indicated. Two to six units of blood should be requested depending upon the severity of the haemorrhage and central venous pressure monitoring considered.

Patients Who Have Delivered Prior to Arrival at the Hospital

Assess clinical condition; arrange theatre for removal of retained placenta.

All Other Abnormalities in Labour

Discuss with registrar.

Cases Requiring Placental Localization or Pelvimetry X-rays

There's little place for pelvimetry X-rays.

Obstetric Operations

Below are given some points in management for obstetric operations.

External Cephalic Version

External cephalic version is now rarely indicated.

Induction of Labour

For all patients having elective inductions and internal monitoring *full aseptic technique and gowning* is indicated. For serial vaginal examinations a *clean* (not gowned) technique is permissible:

i.   Patients for elective induction of labour may receive a cup of tea and toast at 06:15 hours. Enemas may be given pre-induction.
ii. A low amniotomy will be performed if the head is presenting and is engaged. If the head is not engaged, the *registrar should be informed before rupturing the membranes.*
iii. The following regimes are advised:

 a. *Oxytocin*

ARM and Cardiff Pump as required by RMO, or ARM and oxytocin infusion as required by the RMO.

Oxytocin regime

To commence with oxytocin 2 units in D5 solution or 10 units oxytocin in 500 ml of D5 solution.

1st bottle 500 ml (oxytocin 2 units).

20 drops/min for 30 min depending on contractions and then increase by 10 drops/min for 30 min depending on contractions and then increase to a maximum of 60 drops/min until the first 500 ml has been infused.

2nd bottle 500 ml (oxytocin 4 units).

20 drops/min for 30 min depending on contractions and then increase by 10 drops/min every 30 min to a maximum of 60 drops/min.

3rd bottle 500 ml (oxytocin 8 units) on doctor's instructions.

 b. *Prostaglandins*

Prostaglandins may be elected for induction. Potentially they are advantageous in that:

1. They may be administered orally or vaginally.
2. They have no antidiuretic effect.
3. They are effective at all gestations if given in sufficient quantities.
4. They sensitize the uterus to oxytocin.

They suffer from the following disadvantages:
nausea, vomiting, diarrhoea and phlebitis (with intravenous infusions) and they may cause hypertonus and potentiate oxytocin.

Their possible fetal roles include:

1. Intra-uterine fetal death (p. 135).
2. Oral/vaginal prostaglandins + amniotomy for patients with favourable cervices.
3. To sensitize the uterus pre-oxytocin infusion in patients with unfavourable cervices (vaginal pessaries or gel are used).
4. Extra-amniotic route for cases with unfavourable cervices.
5. Necessity for intact membranes.
6. Gross fluid retention or severe pre-eclampsia.

iv. RMOs should do their own elective inductions at 08:00 hours or as early as possible in the morning. Only 'emergency' inductions should be considered at other times.

v. Many patients now attend 'natural childbirth classes' and may decline epidural analgesia or intravenous infusions. The RMO should write in the notes that he/she has offered such facilities, the reasons for so doing and that the patient has declined the same.

Breech Delivery

The merits of vaginal delivery or elective caesarean section should be debated. If vaginal delivery is elected, measurements of biparietal diameter by scanning and pelvic measurements using erect lateral pelvimetry may be used.

Fetal abnormalities should be considered. Breech presentations may be allowed to go into spontaneous labour or be induced at 38–39 weeks' gestation. Epidural analgesia is advisable. A paediatrician and anaesthetist should be present at delivery.

Manual Removal of Placenta
See p. 70.

All Forceps Deliveries
If, at the end of 60 minutes (primigravida) or 30 minutes (multigravida) in the second stage, delivery is not imminent, the RMO must be called.

All Cases of Postpartum Haemorrhage
a. Assistance should be requested.
b. The RMO should commence an intravenous infusion containing 50 IU oxytocin and commence at 5 drops/min for 10 min and increase to 10 drops/min until uterine contractions are palpable.
c. Intravenous ergometrine 0·5 mg should be given.
d. The uterus should be massaged to encourage a uterine contraction.
e. The registrar and theatre should be informed.
f. Two units of blood should be requested.
g. The cause of the haemorrhage should be determined—an examination under anaesthesia will normally be required.
h. A bleeding diathesis, e.g. hypofibrinogenaemia should be considered.
i. The consultant on call should be kept informed.
j. All patients requiring blood transfusion should have a strict fluid balance and vital signs chart.

Whenever a Blood Transfusion is Required

Discuss with registrar.

All Shocked Patients

Consider the cause of shock—hypovolaemic, septicaemic, neurogenic.

Third Degree Tear or Multiple Tears

Repair under general anaesthesia (Chapter 10, p. 99).

All Cases of Torn Cervix

Consider repair under general anaesthesia in theatre.

All Cases of Postpartum Hypertension

Prophylaxis

Restrict ergometrine in labour.

Therapeutic

a. The vital signs should be monitored.

b. Mild sedation with amylobarbitone or diazepam.

c. Initiate renal function tests.

d. The general practitioner should continue the supervision of the patient who is discharged after 48 hours.

e. Arrange a medical outpatient appointment at 6–12 weeks' gestation for further investigations.

All Cases of Suspected Deep Vein Thrombosis

Consider venogram prior to anticoagulation.

Puerperal Pyrexia
Determine cause, consider isolation.

Premature Rupture of the Membranes
If this is confirmed (Ledward and Hawkins, 1983).

Patients with Retained Placenta
Placenta retained *in situ* more than 15 min after delivery of the child.

Definition
When the placenta is still *in situ* more than 15 minutes after delivery of the child.

Procedure
a. Inform registrar.
b. Commence intravenous infusion of normal saline (0·9%).
c. Send serum to the laboratory for cross-matching.
d. Inform the anaesthetist.
e. Under general anaesthesia (or acceptable epidural analgesic) and using aseptic technique, the patient is swabbed and gowned and catheterized. A hand is then placed in the vagina and, using a shearing action, the placenta is separated and withdrawn gently from the uterus. Oxytocin + ergometrine (Syntometrine) 1 ml is given *intravenously* and a gentle curettage of the uterus is performed.
f. If there is no excessive blood loss and no clinical need for a blood transfusion, cancel the request for the cross-match.

g. The obstetrics registrar should ensure that the anaesthetic registrar does *not* wait for the blood to be cross-matched prior to commencing the operation (p. 80).

Prolapsed Cord

a. Assistance should be requested and the RMO and registrar informed.
b. The foot of the bed should be elevated.
c. The presenting part should be held away from the cord per vaginum.
d. The RMO will:
    i.   Commence intravenous infusion.
    ii. Request 2 units of blood.
    iii. Inform theatre.
e. Delivery will be expedited preferably in the theatre.
f. Calm efficiency is preferable to disorganized chaos!

Where Oxytocin is Indicated for Multiparous Patients Who Have Had a Previous Caesarean Section

Fetal and maternal monitoring. Monitor pulse rate.

Any Other Untoward Incident or Anxiety

Inform registrar.

SUMMARY

If in doubt, inform the registrar or consultant!

FURTHER READING
deSwiet M. (1985) Antihypertensive drugs in pregnancy. *Br. Med. J.* **291**, 365–366

HMSO (1986) Guidelines for management of major obstetric haemor-rhage. In: *Report on Confidential Enquiries with Maternal Deaths in England & Wales 1979–81.* London

Ledward R. S. and Hawkins D. F. (1983) *Drug Treatment in Obstetrics.* London, Chapman & Hall

Moir D. D. (1982) *Pain Relief in Labour,* 4th Edn. Edinburgh, Churchill Livingstone

Studd J. (1973) Partograms and nomograms of cervical dilatation in management of primigravida labour. *Br. Med. J.* **4**, 451–455

Vaughan Williams C., Johnson A. and Ledward R. S. (1974) A compari-son of central venous pressure changes in the third stage of labour following oxytoxic drugs and diazepam. *J. Obstet. Gynaecol. Br. Commonw.* **81**, 596–599

Chapter 7

General Practitioner Obstetric Units

INTRODUCTION

General practitioners and community midwife deliveries should be encouraged *within* consultant supervised hospital units. 'Flying squad' calls should be reduced to the minimum.

GUIDELINES FOR OPERATION

General Practitioner Qualification

a. Should be on obstetric list.

b. Should live and practice within the catchment area of the hospital and be able to satisfy the administration committee as to availability.

c. Each GP should nominate a deputy/deputies who should also be on the obstetric list and be a member of a medical defence organization.

d. General practitioners would be required to produce evidence of qualification and membership of a defence organization to the District Management Team on being accepted to use the Unit.

Responsibility

a. The doctor booking a patient for a GP bed will be fully responsible for all antenatal care, confinement and postnatal care, unless he requires consultant advice, in which case a decision will be reached whether transfer to the consultant unit is more appropriate. The GP will be responsible for discharging mother and child, unless transfer to the consultant unit has been arranged. He will ensure that all notes are up to date.

b. The GP obstetrician will be expected to conform with the standard practices and procedures of the obstetric unit.

c. Patients booked for the GP beds may be seen in a consultant clinic at any stage of pregnancy. A visit at 36 weeks may be valuable.

d. The GP will be responsible for conducting the confinement, but the hospital nursing staff will be responsible for 'providing service' after transfer to the postnatal ward, reporting to the general practitioner concerned.

e. The hospital will provide all drugs, sterile supplies etc.

f. Junior medical staff would not normally be involved in the treatment of general practitioner cases, but if circumstances arose in which the midwifery staff considered it imperative to call on the resident junior medical staff, then the patient should automatically be transferred to consultant care.

g. In the case of any complication in labour the duty obstetric registrar should be contacted by the GP when the patient will be transferred to the consultant unit.

Suitable Cases

a. Should be healthy women with no significant obstetric or medical history, aged between 18 and 34 years, above 5 ft in height, and having their second, third or fourth child. There should be a single fetus, with cephalic presentation, and there should be no antibodies and no hydramnios.

b. Higher risk patients may be considered, by agreement with the consultant after referral to the antenatal consultant clinic before 36 weeks.

Administration
a. Referrals for booking in the GP unit are made to the sister in the antenatal clinic. She obtains the mother's medical records and liaises with the district midwife, who will complete the booking forms. When these have been completed, each case is discussed by the committee which normally comprises one consultant gynaecologist and one general practitioner.
b. The patient is fully booked and examined in her own home.

Anticipated Admission
a. The patient would automatically contact her community midwife/GP who would visit her at home and assess the progress of labour.
b. If permissible, the patient may be prepared in her own home, i.e. vulval shave and enema.
c. On deciding that labour is established, the midwife must inform the GP who will arrange for the patient's admission and accompany the patient to hospital.
d. The labour suite must be informed by the midwife of the anticipated arrival.

On Arrival of Patient at the Hospital
a. Case notes will be obtained by receptionist.
b. A delivery room will be allocated and the patient's name entered on room allocation board.
c. Equipment in the delivery room will be available for the use of the midwife.

d. The conduct of labour may be carried out in accordance with the normal procedure of the hospital maternity unit.

e. If any problems arise during the course of labour, the midwife should consult the general practitioner, although in an emergency, the obstetric emergency unit may be consulted, i.e. the consultant on call for that day.

f. It is anticipated that the community midwife will use drugs from the hospital supply, e.g. drugs for pain relief and use of oxytocic drugs (excluding oxytocin, i.e. Syntocinon).

g. In the event of the midwife being called away from the labour suite, e.g. to attend another patient or clinic etc., she should arrange for her colleague to relieve her after consultation with the nursing officer or sister-in-charge. However, coffee and lunch breaks will be covered by the hospital midwife.

EMERGENCY OBSTETRIC SERVICE ('FLYING SQUAD')

Members of Staff

The following *members of staff* could attend flying squad calls:

1. Obstetric consultant or registrar/RMO.
2. Anaesthetic registrar.
3. Medical student.
4. Midwife (if no midwife is at the house) or nurse.
5. Obstetric pupil nurses.

'Flying Squad' Book

The 'flying squad' book contains details of all squad calls and should be completed on return.

'Flying Squad' Equipment

The 'flying squad' equipment should be checked after use and routinely each week by the midwife in charge and the registrar.

Switchboard

When the obstetric 'flying squad' call is received, the call is transferred immediately to the labour suite. Switchboard staff are then alert and ready to receive calls from the labour suite to the ambulance control and obstetric registrar.

Receipt of Call

When the call is received on the labour suite, the midwife will:

a. Note the time, take name, address and telephone number.

b. Ascertain the reason for the call, e.g. APH or PPH, the amount of loss etc.

c. Recall switchboard.
    Transfer the person requesting the flying squad to the obstetric registrar.
    Ask for Ambulance Control giving them precise details and ask the ambulance to go to a prearranged central collecting point.

d. Arrange for blood to be brought to the central collecting point after receiving the registrar's instructions.

e. Take marked box containing pethidine 2 ampoules 100 mg and key ring for the obstetric 'flying squad' cases from the controlled drugs cupboard.

f. Take the box from the labour suite fridge containing:
    Ergometrine
    Ergometrine and oxytocin
    Oxytocin (Syntocinon)

Amyl nitrite

Blood specimen bottles (*see* Appendix IV).

g. Place all equipment on a trolley.

h. Take trolley to the central collecting point to meet the obstetric registrar and ambulance.

Duties of Obstetric Registrar

a. Find out from person requesting flying squad:
- i. Blood group of patient.
- ii. If placenta *in* or *out*.

b. Contact consultant obstetrician on duty.

c. Tell the labour ward midwife what blood is requested:
- i. O Rh negative—2 units ⎫ from refrigerator in
- ii. Correct group—2 units ⎬ pathology laboratory.

d. Collect telephone numbers of pathology technician on call.

e. Go out in the ambulance as soon as possible.

The nearest hospital to the patient's home should take flying squad calls; if the registrar is off-duty the senior house officer (SHO) should contact the consultant obstetrician on call and request advice. If the consultant is not immediately available the SHO should collect the necessary equipment and take this to the patient requesting another SHO or the midwife to contact the consultant. The consultant on duty should always be informed.

No patient suffering from *retained placenta* or postpartum haemorrhage should be moved from their home unless specific directions have been given by the consultant obstetrician on duty.

'PRACTICE RUN'

The obstetric registrar should arrange a practice 'flying squad' twice a year.

FURTHER READING

Chard T. and Richards M. (1977) What do women want? The question of choice in the conduct of labour. In *Benefits and Hazards of the New Obstetrics*, Chap. 4. Ed. E. M. D. Riley. London, Spastics International Medical Publications, William Heinemann Medical Books

Crawford J. S. (1965) Domiciliary practice and flying squad. In *Principles and Practice of Obstetric Anaesthesia,* 2nd edn, Ed. by J. S. Crawford, pp. 340–344. Oxford, Blackwell Scientific

Chapter 8

Obstetric Analgesia and Anaesthesia

INTRODUCTION

This subject is large and covers psychotherapy, hypnosis, regional, local and general anaesthesia and analgesia. Residents in obstetrics should learn to become competent at performing the epidural technique.

BLOOD TRANSFUSIONS

All obstetric patients will have had their blood grouped and, provided there is at least two hours' warning before an emergency caesarean section, two units of blood should have been cross-matched and be present in the theatre before surgery is commenced. If, however, there has been insufficient time to cross-match blood completely, then two units should be requested on a quick cross-match and be sent to the operating theatre as soon as possible. Manual removal of the placenta is another procedure for which two units of blood should be routinely available, but it will always be necessary to have a quick cross-match in these cases.

PRE-OPERATIVE ASSESSMENT

The obstetric houseman should inform the anaesthetist of the proposed list and, after discussion, the anaesthetist will determine whether a pre-operative visit from the anaesthetist will be needed and what pre-medication will be required. If SHOs are required to provide anaesthesia for obstetric cases, the consultant anaesthetist must be informed.

PREPARATION FOR GENERAL ANAESTHETIC

All patients who are to receive a general anaesthetic should have had a history taken and a physical examination before the anaesthetist is informed. Special attention should be paid to the cardiorespiratory systems, and to any anatomical abnormalities of the face, chin, teeth or neck. It is the anaesthetist's duty to see the patient before operation whenever possible and to order the pre-medication that is desired. However, it might be necessary on some occasions for the anaesthetist to request that the obstetric houseman will carry out this visit and pre-medication. The anaesthetist should be notified of a forthcoming operation as soon as possible. However, it is realized that there will be many occasions when there are only a few minutes' interval between the decision to operate and the operation beginning. The anaesthetist is usually requested to 'stand by' in case his assistance is needed during breech deliveries and it would be of particular value if the anaesthetist could be informed of this requirement as soon as possible, rather than at the last moment.

The anaesthetic registrar is encouraged to join the daily labour ward round with the obstetric registrar.

FEEDING IN LABOUR

All mothers who have a high risk of having general anaesthetic, such as those with breech presentation, unstable lie or toxaemia, should be fed entirely by intra-venous fluids throughout labour (Gillett *et al.*, 1984; McAuley *et al.*, 1984; Morgan, 1984).

The principal risk of anaesthesia during labour is from the possibility of inhaling vomit, and because it is the pH of the stomach contents which is the most important single factor in causing subsequent respiratory symptoms, magnesium trisilicate mixture 15 ml is given to each mother in labour every two hours and a further 30 ml is given within half an hour of any proposed general anaesthetic (*see* p. 88).

EPIDURAL ANALGESIA

Explanation to the Patient

The patient should be informed that the pain of con-tractions will be greatly eased but that the perineum may need extra local anaesthetic when the baby is about to be born. The patient may also experience:

i.   Tingling of the skin.
ii. Heaviness and temporary difficulty in moving the legs.
iii. The occasional temporary retention of urine, requiring catheterization.

Contraindications

Contraindications to epidurals include:

i.   Patient resistance.
ii. Local sepsis in lumbar region.
iii. Bleeding or clotting disorders.
iv. Hypotension.
v.   Neurological disease.
vi. Sensitivity to local anaesthetic.

Consent for Epidurals

Epidural analgesia should preferably only be performed at the request of a registrar or more senior obstetrician. However, before the anaesthetist is requested to perform the epidural injection, the procedure should be fully explained to the mother and she should have given her consent. Informed verbal consent is acceptable.

General Management of Epidurals

Midwifery sisters, if approved in technique by the anaesthetists and certified accordingly to comply with Central Midwives Board rules may 'top up' epidurals; special revision lectures should be given on a regular basis.

i.   All patients for epidural will need an intravenous infusion.
ii.   A pre-load of 500 ml Hartman's solution will be given by the anaesthetists at the time of starting the epidural block.
iii.   Mothers must be nursed lying on the side at all times after the epidural is started. Lying flat on the back is forbidden. It allows the uterus to compress the aorta and vena cava and causes a serious reduction in the placental blood flow. It is possible for the placental blood flow to be markedly reduced by aorto–caval compression even though the maternal blood pressure is maintained, or shows only a slight fall.
iv.   The anaesthetist setting up the epidural must give the first dose of local anaesthetic through the catheter. Qualified obstetric nursing staff may give epidural 'top ups' if they have received special instruction, and if they have a properly signed certificate. 'Top ups' will be needed every $1\frac{1}{4}$–3 or 4 hours, depending

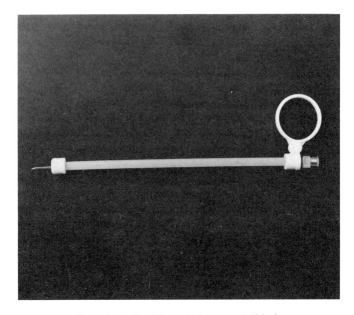

Fig. 8.1. Pudendal needle for pudendal block.

upon the individual patient. As labour progresses, the frequency of 'top ups' increases. The anaesthetist who set up the epidural will specify the volume and strength of the solution needed for 'top ups'. The maximum dose of Marcaine bupivacaine hydrochloride is 2 mg/kg in any four-hour period. The blood pressure must be measured before each 'top up' and at intervals of 5, 10, 15 and 20 minutes afterwards.

If the blood pressure falls the patient may feel sick, faint, dizzy or have ringing in the ears and the mother may look very pale and feel cold.

Systolic levels less than 100 mmHg and systolic falls of more than 25 mmHg from the resting value require

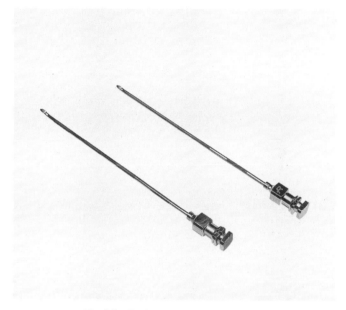

Fig. 8.2. Tuohy needle for epidural block.

treatment. Under these circumstances the anaesthetist must be informed.

vi. During epidural analgesia the mother will have tingling and paraesthesia of the skin and abdomen and legs.

vii. The patient must be turned regularly from side to side and may need help to move.

viii. When an epidural is effective, the sensation of a full bladder is lost, but voiding should be possible before each 'top up', and mothers must be encouraged to try to micturate. If retention of urine occurs, the bladder should be catheterized with full aseptic precautions, and the catheter removed after emptying.

ix.   If a *tap of cerebrospinal fluid* (CSF) occurs during the attempt to set up the epidural, the consultant anaesthetist must be informed: an effective epidural must be done at another intervertebral level. After a CSF tap the labour must be conducted smoothly. There should be no pushing in the second stage. A forceps delivery will be needed. These measures will lessen leakage of CSF from the subarachnoid space, and will reduce the severity of postspinal headache.

x.   Any severe headache occurring in the postpartum period must be notified to the consultant anaesthetist as prompt treatment will help.

xi.   Assessment of the approach of the second stage is more difficult in epidural cases as the bearing down reflex may be lost or modified, so vaginal examination may be needed at more frequent intervals to check progress of labour.

xii. During the second stage the mother should be able to cooperate with pushing as instructed and encouraged by her obstetric attendants. Only infrequently will the motor-block from the epidural be so complete that pushing down is not at all possible. However, the incidence of 'lift-out forceps' is increased by epidurals.

xiii. The epidural catheter should normally be removed immediately after delivery by a midwife who should sign the epidural form to confirm that the catheter was intact.

The epidural catheter may be left in place for pain relief after caesarean section.

Complications of Epidurals

There are two serious complications of epidurals. These are respiratory paralysis of the mother and maternal hypotension.

Respiratory Paralysis

Respiratory paralysis is very rare and can *always* be treated successfully with no permanent harm to the mother providing the attending staff act correctly. All staff dealing with patients having epidurals must be confident in their own minds that they could properly ventilate and oxygenate an epidural patient who stopped breathing. Ventilatory assistance would mean passing a plastic airway and using a face-mask with an Ambubag to blow air into the lungs. Remember that such a paralysed epidural patient would be fully conscious. Encourage and reassure the patient.

Maternal Hypotension

Maternal hypotension must be treated if the blood pressure falls to below 100 mmHg systolic, or if there is a fall greater than 25 mmHg from the resting value. A doctor must be informed.

Maternal hypotension may reduce the placental blood flow and there may be abnormalities in the fetal heart rate. The patient must be on her side. Sometimes lying on one particular side maintains blood pressure better than when on the other side. Further amounts of intravenous fluid may be needed. Ephedrine by intravenous injections, 6 mg increments should be given every two minutes, timed by a clock, up to a mximum of 3 doses. If these measures do not restore the blood pressure within 10 minutes, then more experienced advice must be obtained immediately.

COMPLICATED OBSTETRIC CASES

Breech, Trial of Labour, Multiple Pregnancy etc.

The anaesthetist should be forewarned prior to the second stage of labour; blood should preferably be cross-matched.

Retained Placentae

Patients should have blood taken for cross-match and then be taken to theatre whilst the blood is being prepared; it is impossible to wait several hours for the blood to be ready since (i) it may not be required, (ii) the patient may bleed heavily in the interim if the placenta is kept *in situ*. Appropriate uncross-matched blood must be used if it becomes necessary before the cross-matched blood arrives.

Emergency Cases in Need of Transfusions

The safety of the mother is the primary concern, e.g.:

i.   If blood is not available, the decision to operate must be made by the consultant staff (but *see above*).

ii. If the obstetrician wishes to proceed but the junior anaesthetist has reservations, the case should be discussed with the consultant anaesthetic staff.

CAESAREAN SECTION (*See also* p. 102)

i.   The patient should be properly assessed pre-operatively.

ii.   Planned caesarean section patients will have been fasting for 12 hours pre-operatively.

iii. Pre-medication should be with 1 ml metoclopromide 10 mg 45 min pre-operatively and 15 ml oral 0·3 M sodium citrate, just as the patient leaves the ward to go to the theatre. (Ranitidine hydrochloride, 150 mg, may be used instead of sodium citrate.) Metoclopromide promotes gastric emptying and may increase the tone in the lower oesophageal sphincter and lessens the chances of regurgitation.

Atropine decreases the tone in the lower oesophageal sphincter and should not be used.

An effective buffer is 15 ml 0·3 M sodium citrate.

(Magnesium trisilicate mixture has recently been implicated as a causative agent in aspiration-pneumonitis if it gets into the lungs.)

iv.   The mother should be taken to the theatre lying with the right side downwards. This will promote gastric emptying. It will also reduce aorto–caval compression by the uterus.

v..   Induction of anaesthesia should be done in the theatre on the operating table.

vi.   One or preferably two members of the theatre staff should be designated to assist the anaesthetist.

vii. Pre-oxygenation and cricoid pressure are to be used in every case.

viii. All patients must have a freely running intravenous infusion before the induction of anaesthesia.

ix.   Cross-matched compatible whole blood should be available before the start of the anaesthetic. If blood is not available the consultant anaesthetist must be informed.

x.   Obstetric anaesthetics should not be given by anaesthetists with less than 1 years' experience in the specialty.

xi.   An experienced paediatrician should attend the operation to resuscitate the baby if needed.

FURTHER READING

Gillett G. B., Watson J. D. and Langford R. M. (1984) Ranitidine and single-dose antacid therapy as prophylaxis against acid aspiration syndrome in obstetric practice. *Anaesthesia*, **39**, 638–644

McAuley D. M., Moore J., Dundee J. W. and McCaughey W. (1984) Oral ranitidine in labour. *Anaesthesia*, **39**, 433–438

Morgan M. (1984) Control of intragastric pH and volume. *Br. J. Anaesth.* **56**, 47

Waldron B. A. (1983) *Management of Epidural Analgesia in Childbirth*, 2nd edn. London, Churchill Livingstone

Chapter 9

The Postnatal Ward

INTRODUCTION

The postnatal involvement by medical staff can be dangerously ignored and yet remains a major part of care. It tends to be delegated to supervision by postnatal midwives and residents with registrar and consultant involvement being minimal.

This 'fourth stage of labour' phase varies in time and may be anything from 6 hours to a 10-day postpartum stay, but most multigravid mothers tend to be discharged after 48 hours, which would appear to be a reasonable compromise to ensure no major problem arises, to allow the mother appropriate and reasonable rest, to allow midwife supervision in the establishment of breast feeding and to allow time for medical (obstetric and paediatric) supervision of mother and baby.

When patients are discharged from home the community midwife has a legal obligation to continue supervision of mother and child for a period of 28 days and the postnatal clinic consultation should normally be undertaken by the patient's general practitioner except for complicated deliveries (*see below*) where the patient should be seen at the consultant's postnatal clinic at 6-weeks postpartum.

Postnatal wards at present are normally clinically designed units and should probably continue to be so, but rooms could be available to allow a more 'natural' environment for those patients who may be totally averse to hospital delivery or postnatal care.

The registrar and resident medical officer should undertake a daily ward round of the postnatal ward and the major duties of the RMO include the duties listed below.

INVESTIGATIONS

Haematology

Check that all mothers have blood taken for haemoglobin estimation on the third day, or prior to discharge in the case of early discharge patients; a further haemoglobin check should be done by the community midwife.

Check that cord and maternal blood have been taken in all cases where the mother is rhesus negative. Check the result of these investigations and check that anti-D serum has been given within 72 hours of delivery where warranted. Also check that the record form and cooperation card have been filled in after administration of anti-D (see p. 158). Anti-D should be given to rhesus negative patients in the puerperium, following a miscarriage or following external cephalic version.

See that rhesus negative mothers with antibodies have blood taken for antibody titre at the appropriate time as directed by the laboratory.

Microbiology

Ensure that patients with obvious evidence of infection are transferred to single rooms.

Examine all patients with a pyrexia of 38°C or over and see that a mid-stream specimen of urine and high vaginal swab are taken for culture and sensitivity. Exclude deep vein thrombosis/pulmonary embolism or breast abcess.

Ensure that a repeat mid-stream specimen of urine is sent for microscopy and culture and sensitivity prior to discharge of any mother who has had a urinary tract infection during pregnancy.

Check that rubella vaccination is given if indicated.

PERINEAL DISCOMFORT

Ultrasound Therapy

The effects of insonation are localized generation of heat, micro-massage in depth, biological reactions including analgesia and inhibition of inflammatory (non-bacterial) processes. For treating perineal bruising, insonate for 5 minutes using a conducting medium (gel, water baths or water pillows), with a 3–4 cm diameter transducer head travelling over the area affected. The dose varies according to the severity of the bruising and patient tolerance.

Usually there is lessening of swelling and some analgesia after the first treatment and, certainly by the third, a marked improvement is apparent.

Ultrasonic treatment for bruising and haematomas after caesarean sections is also very beneficial.

SUPPRESSION OF LACTATION

This should be treated if indicated. Painful, engorged breasts may be a cause of puerperal pyrexia and treatment with analgesia (aspirin) and supportive bras will normally be all that will be required. However, occasionally, for example where the patient has had a stillborn or neonatal death, the use of bromocriptine 2·5 mg twice a day for 14 days may be advocated. This preparation is relatively expensive and there is little place for its routine use for patients who elect not to breast feed.

CONTRACEPTION

This specific aspect of the postnatal management provides par excellence an example of departmental discussion with individual registrars, consultants (obstetricians and paediatricians), general practitioners, and patients and will vary from unit to unit.

The subject may have been mentioned at some stage during the antenatal period and many patients will have elected their appropriate form of contraception. Other patients are happy to discuss contraception during the immediate puerperium whilst others prefer to discuss the subject with their own general practitioner at the postnatal clinic.

If oral contraception has been chosen in the absence of specific contraindications, it is not unreasonable to commence a low dose combined oestrogen–progesterogen pill (containing less than 50 μg oestrogen) from the day of discharge from hospital. Such an approach will provide contraception, help reduce lochia, help involution and provide the patient with an indication of date of her first menstrual period. Most authorities do not believe that breast feeding is suppressed with the use of combined oestrogen–progestogen preparations.

Barrier methods of contraception or intra-uterine contraceptives may be elected.

The subject of sterilization may have been discussed during the antenatal period and an elective procedure arranged. This is best undertaken on an elective date at 3–6 months postpartum by laparoscopy. Breast feeding mothers can be accommodated on a day case or overnight stay basis. Rarely, puerperal sterilization using the Pomeroy technique may be advised, but in view of the added risk of deep vein thrombosis it is more usual to defer the sterilization procedure.

Sterilization should be considered as a permanent procedure and it is unreasonable to ask the patient if she would like sterilization procedure immediately before a caesarean section; however, it is not unreasonable to perform a sterilization procedure during a caesarean section provided both parents have discussed the arguments for and against the procedure during the relative calm of the antenatal period.

The case for an elective sterilization procedure on a date

3–6 months postpartum allows time for both partners to be absolutely certain of their wishes and ensures no immediate neonatal catastrophe has arisen.

The procedures available are numerous (*see* p. 106).

EXPLANATION TO MOTHER

Ensure that mothers understand the nature of any medical procedure that has been or is being carried out on them and the nature of any abnormality their baby suffers from, provided that the diagnosis is certain.

DISCHARGE FROM HOSPITAL

Occasionally, patients decide to leave hospital prior to the time previously arranged with their consultant. This may be due to social problems. The RMO should encourage the patient to stay, but otherwise the patient should sign the 'Discharge against Medical Advice' form. The GP and community midwife should then be informed.

Early Discharge

Instructions for discharge should be given to those patients booked for early discharge who are free to go (a minimum of 24 hours after delivery). Check that the community midwife found the home situation suitable and is able to accept the patient.

General Assessment

A general assessment and examination of the patient should be made prior to discharge including:

a. Vital physical signs.

b. Breast examination.

c. Abdominal examination.

d. Perineal examination including examination of episiotomy sutures.

e. A vaginal examination should be within normal limits and no excessive loss evident.

f. No evidence of deep vein thrombosis should be present.

g. Residents should be alert to the possibility of psychosis developing in the postpartum patient. The 'Fourth Day Blues' are acceptable, but pathological psychosis merits further therapy.

Discharge Letter

The midwife gives the patient a discharge letter and this is handed to the district midwife. A letter is posted direct to the general practitioner. Cooperation cards are completed by the midwife.

Complete Discharge Summaries Within 24 Hours of Discharge

It is the responsibility of the obstetric or paediatric RMO to examine newborn babies and to be responsible for the care of those remaining only 48 hours in the unit. It is the responsibility of the paediatric RMO after the initial examination to be responsible for those remaining in the unit for more than 48 hours and for the *final examination* before the baby goes home.

After discharge

Occasionally, once the patient has been discharged, problems may arise and the general practitioner may request a readmission; in such cases an immediate re-admission for reassessment should be arranged and examples include:

a. Perineum breakdown—as long as the perineum is clear there is little place for a repeat surgical repair and the perineum will normally heal perfectly within 6 weeks.
b. Pulmonary embolism—review with medical colleagues should be arranged.
c. Postpartum haemorrhage.
d. Puerperal sepsis.

POSTNATAL CLINIC APPOINTMENTS

These are normally undertaken by the patients' general practitioner at 6-weeks postpartum. However, where complications have arisen the patient should be asked to attend the hospital postnatal clinics for assessment and discussion with the registrar and consultants in the cases of, for example:

a. Caesarean section.
b. Difficult and traumatic vaginal deliveries.
c. Prolonged labour.
d. Unexplained stillborn or neonatal death.
e. Major medical and surgical complications.
f. If in doubt, or if the patient requests a hospital postnatal consultation.
g. If an intra-uterine contraceptive device has been elected and the patient requests this to be undertaken by a hospital clinic (alternatives include the general practitioner or family planning clinic).

SUMMARY

The postnatal ward is '*par excellence*', the RMO's 'empire'; the puerperium should be considered the fourth stage of labour and given serious supervision by the RMO.

FURTHER READING

Passmore C. M., McElnay J. C. and D'Arcy P. F. (1984) Drugs taken by mothers in the puerperium inpatient survey in Northern Ireland. *Br. Med. J.* **289**, 1593

Swyer G. (1985) Postpartum mental disturbances and hormone changes. *Br. Med. J.* **290**, 1232–1233

Chapter 10

Surgical Procedures

OBSTETRIC SURGERY

Introduction

The resident medical officer in obstetrics will be required to be competent at:

a. Episiotomy and episiorrhaphy; repair of third and fourth degree tears (p. 99).
b. Management of retained placenta (p. 70).
c. Evacuation of retained products of conception (p. 101).
d. Caesarean section (p. 102).
e. Sterilization (p. 106).

The resident will be responsible for arranging post-partum operating lists and should ensure:

a. Consent forms are signed (the husband's consent is not legally required for sterilization procedures). Puerperal sterilization procedures are not now encouraged in view of the potential risk of associated deep vein thrombosis. Interval laparoscopic procedures are advisable.
b. The patient has been reminded of the full consequences of the procedure.
c. That the operating list has been arranged and that he has informed the anaesthetist, theatre, requested blood for haemoglobin and 'group and save'.
d. He should confirm that histological specimens are sent to the laboratory.

Procedures

Episiotomy and Episiorrhaphy

Alternatives available include (*see Fig.* 10.1).

a. Right mediolateral episiotomy.
b. Midline episiotomy.
c. J-shaped episiotomy.

Absorbable sutures are used for the procedure.

The Technique of Repair of Third or Fourth Degree Lacerations

Definition

1° = perineal laceration.
2° = perineal body torn.
3° = anal sphincters torn.
4° = rectum torn.

Third degree lacerations may be repaired by the RMO, but only after the technique has been taught and demonstrated to him. He must be supervised, until fully competent, by the registrar.

All fourth degree lacerations must be sutured by the registrar; general anaesthesia should be considered.

A suggested approach is:

a. The rectal mucosa is approximated by a continuous Lembert suture of fine catgut, avoiding any penetration into the lumen. This suture starts above the apex of the tear and ends at the mucocutaneous junction.
b. The pre-rectal fascia is sutured over the rectal wound extending down to include the fascia underlying the external anal sphincter. (The anal canal is now reconstituted.)

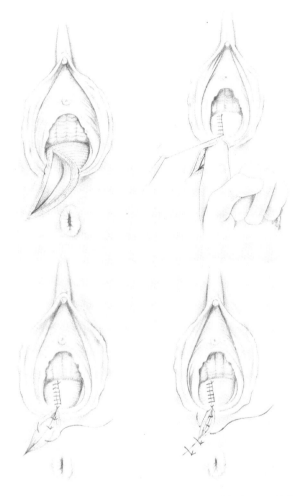

Fig. 10.1. (*a*) Right mediolateral episiotomy; (*b*) closure of the posterior vaginal wall using continuous-lock suture; (*c*) suture of the perineal body muscle with interrupted stitches; (*d*) closure of the skin using interrupted stitches.

c. The external anal sphincter edges are carefully approximated with two or three sutures of thicker catgut (0).

d. The vaginal epithelium is next sewn with continuous fine catgut down to the hymenal ring, again taking care that the first stitch is above the apex of the tear.

e. The deep perineal muscles are now approximated with one, two or three interrupted sutures of the thicker catgut.

f. The final stitch (of fine catgut) starts at the hymenal ring, leaving a long end; it is continuous, running along the superficial perineal muscles, right back and including the fascia covering the external anal sphincter and then by turning the needle and running a subcuticular layer in reverse direction, the skin edges are approximated. The end of the suture is tied inside the vagina to the strand left long at the beginning. Thus, there is no external knot on the perineum and no exposed suture material. The corrugated skin on the anal canal is not sutured because these edges are automatically held together by the sphincter and sutures to this area are unsatisfactory and uncomfortable.

g. The wound is covered with a dry sterile pad and no other dressing is used.

POST-OPERATIVE No special management is required; a hospital postnatal appointment should be given and advice on future deliveries in hospital provided.

Evacuation of the Retained Products of Conception

a. The RMO should request an ultrasound to determine if retained products are *in situ*.

b. If there is evidence of infection, antibiotic cover should be given for 12 hours prior to curettage.

c. Theatre should be informed.

d. The anaesthetist should be informed.

e. Blood should be requested for a haemoglobin as well as 'group and save' serum.

f. Consent for surgery should be obtained.

g. The registrar should be informed.

h. In theatre under general anaesthesia the patient should be swabbed, gowned and catheterized. An examination under anaesthesia should be performed and, using manual dexterity, the excess products of conception removed. The anterior lip of the cervix should be held with a sponge holder and using forceps and a curette the uterus emptied. Oxytocin + ergometrine (Syntometrine) 1 ml should be given or oxytocin by intravenous infusion if ergometrine is contraindicated.

The products should be sent in saline for karyotyping and in formalin for histology.

If the uterus is inadvertently perforated during curettage an immediate laparoscopy will be required to be undertaken by the registrar.

Caesarean section

See Fig. 10.2.

The RMO will be required to:

a. Obtain a duly signed consent form.

b. Inform the parents of the indication for surgery.

c. Inform the anaesthetist and discuss whether a general or epidural anaesthetic will be used.

d. Obtain blood for a haemoglobin and cross-match 2 units of blood.

e. Inform the paediatrician.

f. Determine whether the patient wishes a sterilization procedure to be performed at the time of surgery (p. 106).

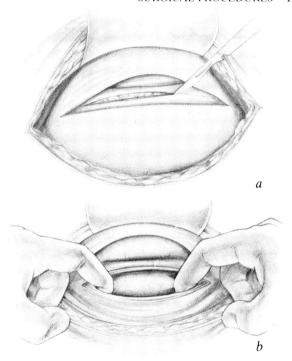

Fig. 10.2. Caesarian section. Operation is performed with patient in supine position. After catheterization of urinary bladder the area of abdomen below the umbilicus is cleaned and draped. Some obstetricians may prefer to leave the catheter *in situ* during the whole operative procedure. (*a*) Exposure of the lower uterine segment through Pfannenstiel or lower midline incision. Doyen's retractor *in situ*. Peritoneal fold is incised with scissors and lower uterine segment opened with scalpel. (*b*) The incision is completed by index fingers extending it laterally. (*c*) Delivery of the child's head after rupturing the membranes. (*d*) Delivery of the placenta by gentle traction following an intravenous dose of oxytocic drug. (*e*) Incision angles secured with single sutures. First layer closure of the lower uterine segment with continuous suture involving half a thickness of the incision. (*f*) Closure completed by suturing the second layer with continuous suture. (*g*) Closure of peritoneum with continuous suture.

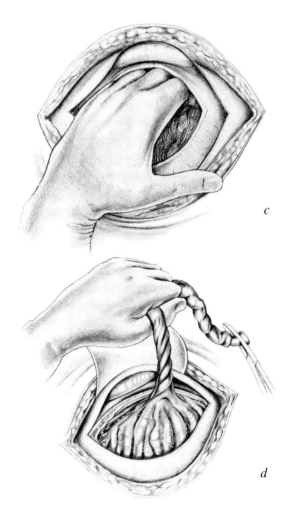

c

d

Fig. 10.2.

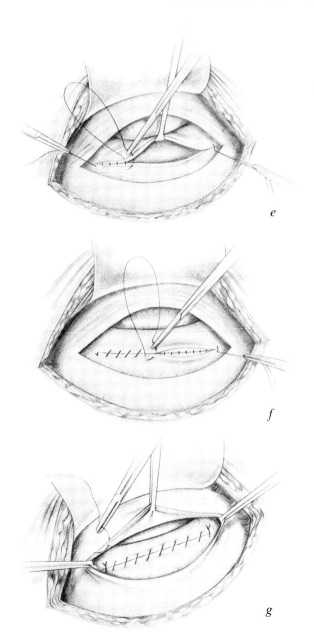

e

f

g

Sterilization

Many methods are available so the indications and procedures should be determined on the basis of local preference.

Possible methods of sterilization include:

a. *Tubal ligation and/or division*
   Varying methods include Pomeroy, Madlener, Uchida and Irving.

   Pomeroy: involves pulling up a loop of the uterine tube, ligating it in two places and excising a portion of loop between the ligatures.

   Madlener: here a loop of tube is pulled up and the loop ligated after crushing the tube with forceps but not excising the tube.

   Uchida: the tube is divided and the uterine end of the tube is buried in the mesosalpinx while the lateral end opens into the peritoneal cavity.

   Irving: each tube is divided and the proximal end is buried in the wall of the uterus through a small puncture site. The distal end is buried in the mesosalpinx.

b. *Aldridge method:* the tubes are not divided but the fimbrian ends are buried in the broad ligament.

c. *Fimbriectomy:* the distal portion of each tube which is vital for ovum transport is excised.

d. *Tubal diathermy:* normally used in conjunction with the laparoscopy using bipolar electric current.

e. *Occlusive bands or rings:* termed 'Yoon bands' or 'Falope rings'; a loop of isthmic portion of the tube is grasped and a small silastic band is placed over the loop, making it avascular.

f. *Laparoscopic interval sterilization* by tubal diathermy occlusive clips (*see Fig.* 10.3) (Filshie, 1986) or silastic rings.

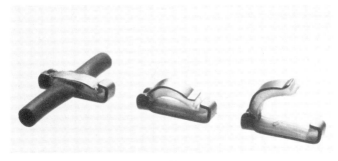

a

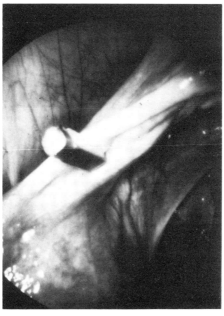

b

Fig. 10.3. (*a*) Titanium Filshie clip; (*b*) Filshie clip *in situ*.

MEDICAL RECORDS

A major, and often neglected, part of the RMO's duty is involved in keeping adequate notes and records. Hospital files may become disorderly and, whilst ward clerks may be available to keep the notes reasonably tidy, the RMO should contribute to ensure that required investigations are undertaken and that abnormal results are filed. Visual display charts should be encouraged so that results may be assessed at intervals.

The RMO should ensure that discharge summaries are kept up-to-date so that the general practitioner is kept fully informed regarding his patients' in-patient care.

All doctors should remain alert to the medico-legal complications of poorly maintained notes.

SUMMARY

The RMO should quickly learn the minor surgical procedures and progress to more major operations.

FURTHER READING

Filshie G. M. (1981) The titanium/silicone rubber clip for female sterilization. *Br. J. Obstet. Gynaecol.* **88**, 655–62.

Rob C. and Smith R. (1976) In: *Operative Surgery, Gynaecology and Obstetrics.* Ed. D. W. T. Roberts. London, Butterworths.

PART II

Neonatology

Chapter 11

Neonatology: Special Care Baby Unit

INTRODUCTION

Ideally the duty obstetrical resident would always contact the neonatal paediatric resident on call for the labour ward and discuss cases where a paediatrician may be needed after delivery. In an emergency, the sister-in-charge or her deputy should call the paediatrician. The paediatric resident should always be available to attend deliveries at the discretion of the obstetrician.

CONDITIONS FOR WHICH PAEDIATRICIANS WOULD ALWAYS BE EXPECTED TO BE CALLED

1. Caesarean section.
2. Breech delivery.
3. Multiple pregnancy.
4. Instrumental delivery:
   Ventouse extraction.
   All forceps deliveries.
5. Pre-term delivery—36 weeks' gestation or less.
6. Fetal distress (as assessed by obstetrician).
7. Severe pregnancy induced hypertension and pre-eclampsia.
8. Maternal diabetes mellitus.
9. Rhesus incompatibility if the fetus is thought to be moderately or severely affected—liaison between the

obstetrician and paediatrician is indicated prior to surgical induction of labour.
10. APH is associated with fetal distress or suspected fetal bleed.
11. Maternal thyrotoxicosis.
12. Maternal myasthenia gravis.
13. Maternal narcotic addiction.
14. Cyanotic heart disease in mother (usually associated with large-for-date infant).
15. If there is doubt about the condition of the baby.

RESUSCITATION OF THE NEWBORN

An adequate airway must be maintained and oral suction alone is normally all that is required. If resuscitation is slow, as evidenced by poor tone and colour of the baby, endotracheal intubation, suction and oxygen will be required and every resident and midwife should be trained in this procedure. Warmth is essential and aluminium foil blankets are mandatory. If the patient has received recent respiratory depressant drugs then antagonism may be required, using naloxone.

MANAGEMENT OF THE NEWBORN BABY IN THE LABOUR WARD

In the labour ward all mothers should be encouraged to hold babies for as long as possible and to put them to the breast if wanting to breast feed. No supplements or glucose etc. should be given in the labour ward or postnatal unit until it is known if mother is breast feeding. The possibilities of unacceptable heat loss with small or premature babies should be remembered.

AVOIDANCE OF UNDUE HEAT LOSS TO NEWBORN BABY IN THEATRE

The temperature in the operating theatre should be turned up and air conditioning turned off before delivery. Great care should be taken, especially with low-birth-weight babies to keep them covered and out of draughts. Hats should be placed on the babies as soon as possible to minimize heat loss from the head.

INFORM THE PAEDIATRIC RMO AFTER DELIVERY

The paediatric RMO should be informed in cases of:

1. Low-birth-weight infants ($<2\cdot5$ kg).
2. Prolonged rupture of membranes (>48 hours).
3. Major congenital abnormalities (minor abnormalities, e.g. digits, may wait until morning).
4. Polyhydramnios if *any* doubt about oesophageal atresia.
5. Previous abnormal infant or perinatal death.
6. Any illness in the mother which may cause problems to the neonate, e.g. idiopathic thrombocytopenic purpura. This should include maternal infection, e.g. tuberculosis, gonorrhoea.
7. Infants who have not established regular respiration.

INDICATIONS FOR ADMISSION TO SPECIAL CARE BABY UNIT

Contact the paediatrician on duty for the special care baby unit before transferring any infant.

The paediatrician who attends the deliveries mentioned above will assess the baby and decide whether or not special care is needed. The aim is to return babies to their mothers as soon as possible.

Admit directly from the labour ward, or immediately after delivery elsewhere:

1. Infants under 2500 g or 35 weeks' gestation.
2. Babies with severe perinatal asphyxia.
3. Babies with respiratory difficulty and/or cyanosis.
4. Babies with serious congenital abnormality.
5. Babies with haemolytic disease.
6. Babies having had a difficult (traumatic) delivery.
7. Babies with maternal illness likely to affect the child, e.g. diabetes, thyrotoxicosis.
8. Babies with previous unexplained neonatal deaths—if previous baby died soon after delivery.
9. Babies for adoption (occasionally).
10. Post-caesarean section babies.
11. Post-general anaesthesia babies.

CONDITIONS OF THE INFANT REQUIRING TRANSFER FROM OUTLYING HOSPITALS

1. Infants under 1500 g.
2. Infants who may require respiratory support.
3. Infants who may require exchange transfusion.
4. Infants who may require surgery.
5. Convulsions, apnoeic or cyanotic attacks.
6. Bleeding.
7. Vomiting.
8. Persistent poor feeding.
9. Infection, if intensive care facilities needed (e.g. septicaemia).
10. On request of GP or midwife.

FURTHER READING

Black J. (1974) *Neonatal Emergencies and Other Problems.* London, Butterworths.

PART III

Gynaecology

Chapter 12

Outpatient Clinics

INTRODUCTION

The patient attending the gynaecological outpatient department may have been assessed by the general practitioner and referred for further investigations. Most patients will be seen by the consultant in charge of the clinic, but occasionally the RMO or registrar will be the second tier of consultation with appropriate referral to the consultant after initial assessment.

HISTORY

A full gynaecological history should be taken including past obstetric, medical and surgical history. Medication should be noted and full details relating to contraception recorded together with the date of the last cervical smear.

EXAMINATION

A general and pelvic examination should include recording the patient's weight, blood pressure, neurological system (for multiple sclerosis), pelvic findings and possibly colposcopic examination of the cervix (normally reserved for patients with positive cervical smear results).

INVESTIGATIONS

These will relate to the presenting symptoms. Outpatient investigations should be as full as possible to reduce possible in-patient assessment.

a. Haemoglobin and blood group. ⎫
b. Full blood count.   ⎬ In most cases
c. Chest X-ray.   ⎭
d. Intravenous urogram.
e. Micturating cystogram.
f. Cervical smear (*Fig.* 12.1).
g. Mid-stream specimen of urine.
h. Cervical swab.
i. Endocrinological studies for amenorrhoea.
j. Ultrasound of pelvic organs (p. 187).

Further Special Investigations

Special investigations may be considered where indicated:

a. Bladder pressure studies (refer to regional centre if not available locally).
b. Colposcopy.
c. Hormonal assays etc.

These tests are expensive and requests should be selective, for examples, *see below*.

Amenorrhoea (p. 142)

It is important to note that (i) Many types of medication interfere with hormone production or with assay methods, and so can give rise to misleading results. All medication must be stated on the request form including any that has been discontinued during the past three or four weeks.

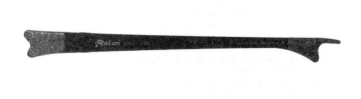

Fig. 12.1. Spatula suitable for cervical smear.

(ii) False results will be obtained unless the sampling conditions described are carefully observed.

PREGNANCY TESTS Tests for β-human chorionic gonadotrophin are of questionable value. Ultrasonography is preferable for confirmation of pregnancy.

CHROMOSOMES AND BUCCAL SMEAR PERFORMED BY THE CYTOLOGY DEPARTMENT (CYTOGENETIC SERVICES)

a. Buccal smears, preliminary test for sex chromosome abnormalities: squamous cells are scraped from the buccal cavity of the mouth and spread onto microscope slides: 6–8 slides are required. They are rapidly fixed in alcohol and stained with 1% cresyl fast violet. A minimum of 200 cells are examined for the presence/absence of Barr bodies and reported as a percentage.

b. Lymphocyte cultures for chromosomal analysis: prepared culture bottles are inoculated with 0·3 ml of venous blood and incubated at 37 °C. The lymphocytes are harvested after 72 hours and cells in metaphase are examined and photographed for karyotyping. Results are normally available in one week.

URINARY 17-OXOSTEROIDS (OR 17-KETOSTEROIDS) AND 17-HYDROXYCORTICOSTEROIDS At least two, preferably three, accurate 24-hour urine collections are required. Pass urine into the toilet at 08:00; thereafter all urine goes into the bottle including that passed exactly at 08:00 next morning. A plain bottle, no preservative, obtainable from the laboratory and returnable.

Specimens must get to the laboratory within two days of collection for valid results. Reporting time 7–10 days.

PITUITARY GONADOTROPHINS

a. Serum LH and FSH: 5 ml clotted blood—no special timing or patient preparation but specimens must reach laboratory before 15:00 on day of taking. Reporting time about 10 days.
b. Urinary LH: 24-hour collection into bottle containing 10 ml of 2% boric acid. Remember to request bottle with boric acid in. Reporting time about 10 days.

PROLACTIN Eight millilitres clotted blood—take in morning when levels show least variation (09:00–12:00). Venepuncture must be successful at first attempt as levels are easily affected by stress. Reporting time 7–10 days.

DYNAMIC FUNCTION TESTS These tests require careful supervision of specimens and must be arranged with the laboratory several days beforehand even if the doctor is going to take his/her own specimens.

a. Gonadotrophic releasing hormone (LHRH) stimulation test: can be done in outpatients or at local hospitals by medical staff (technical staff do not do these tests). Takes about 1·5 hours. Reporting time about 10 days.

b. Oestradiol-17β: arrange beforehand as plasma must be separated without delay. No special timing or patient preparation necessary apart from this; 5 ml blood into heparin. Reporting time about 2 weeks.

c. Testosterone: no special patient preparation or timing required; 5 ml blood into lithium heparin tube and send to laboratory, with request form, at once. Reporting time about 2 weeks.

Laboratory Tests for Other Conditions Sometimes Giving Rise to Amenorrhoea

The usual laboratory tests are available for Cushing's syndrome, Addison's disease, congenital adrenal hyperplasia, malabsorption, thyroid disease, renal failure, diabetes, tuberculosis, connective tissue disorders.

MANAGEMENT OF INDIVIDUAL CASES

Based on findings from the history and investigations, a preliminary diagnosis should be offered for discussion with the consultant together with a plan of management. Outpatient surgery, including cryocautery (*see Fig.* 12.2), vabra aspiration, and insertion of contraceptive devices may be performed.

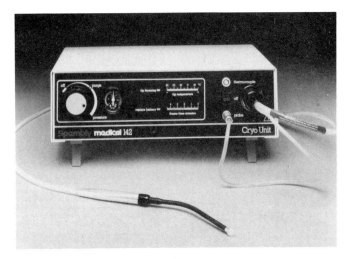

a

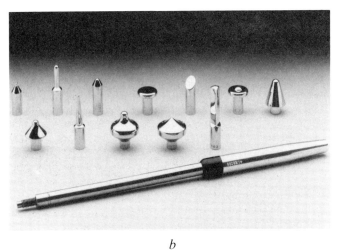

b

Fig. 12.2. (*a*) Cryosurgery unit; (*b*) cryosurgical probes.

FOLLOW-UP CLINIC VISITS

Further visits should be kept to a minimum (*see Table* 12.1), so as to prevent clinic congestion, thus allowing extra time for detailed complicated cases.

Table 12.1. Outpatient follow-up appointments

Symptom	Appointment
Dysfunctional bleeding/ infertility patients	3-month appointment
Major surgery	6-week appointment
Cone biopsy	3-week appointment
Termination/sterilization	Appointment with general practitioner or hospital at 6 weeks
Malignant cases	Every 3 months for 1 year
	Every 6 months for 2 years
	Every 12 months for 3 years
	Every 24 months for 5 years and when indicated

GENITOURINARY MEDICINE

Sexually transmitted diseases are now the commonest group of communicable diseases in the world and the number of infected patients continues to rise every year. The increase in incidence has taken place despite improvements in diagnosis and effective antibiotics which make patients rapidly non-infectious and cure the majority. In recent years, it has become apparent that the number of diseases which are spread by the sexual route is much larger than had been appreciated in the past. In the majority of hospital clinics only a minority of patients are found to be suffering from the older, classical, well-recognized venereal diseases (syphilis and gonorrhoea) and the majority of patients have conditions such as non-specific genital infection, trichomoniasis, candidiasis, genital warts, herpes, molluscum contagiosum, scabies, pediculosis pubis and a variety of other diseases (*Table* 12.2) which have only been recognized as sexually transmissible in recent years. In addition, many patients are found to have other genital conditions which may not be transmitted sexually, as well as psychological, psychosexual and other problems for which they may need the help and advice of an experienced doctor.

Table 12.2. Sexually transmitted diseases

Organism	Disease
Bacteria	Gonorrhoea
	Chancroid
	Granuloma inguinale
Viruses	Non-specific genital infection
	Chlamydial infection
	Herpes genitalis
	Genital warts
	Lymphogranuloma venereum
	Molluscum contagiosum
	Hepatitis B
	AIDS (acquired immune deficiency syndrome)
Spirochaetes	Syphilis
	Balanitis
Protozoa	Trichomoniasis
Fungi	Candidiasis
	Tinea cruris
Parasites	Scabies
	Pediculosis pubis

Slowly it has become apparent that not only are many other diseases passed on by sexual activity, but also the term 'venereal disease' is not entirely satisfactory to describe this group of conditions, because it frequently carries with it an implication of criticism and censure. This is illustrated by the fact that clinics for the treatment of veneral diseases are still frequently hidden away in inaccessible parts of hospitals, are often called 'special clinics' and the patients are sometimes not addressed by name but by number in the mistaken belief that this will hide their identity.

Recent changes in attitude in sexual matters in general and to the sexually transmitted diseases in particular have rendered these arrangements unsatisfactory and the modern outlook is to place clinics in the main outpatients' departments and to treat the patients attending them in exactly the same way as patients attending any other medical clinic in the hospital.

The clinics are supervised by the consultant trained in genitourinary medicine. Trained nurses of both sexes form an important part of the clinic team. Nurses are also trained in contact tracing which forms a very important part of the service. All patients have free access to the clinics and can attend of their own accord without a letter from their general practitioner.

It is important to remember that patients with sexually transmitted diseases have been infected by somebody else and if they are promiscuous they have infected others afterwards. It is essential that all those who may be infected should attend a clinic for examination and treatment. Frequently a contact slip, which is a small piece of paper with the patient's reference number and the diagnosis, is given to the patient and he or she is asked to give this to their contact who is asked to attend the clinic for examination. Failure to carry out contact tracing leads to the spread of infection and often the reinfection of the original patients.

Collection of Specimen for Routine Bacteriology (p. 165)

a. Swab from vagina, cervix and urethra, spread on a clean dry glass slide, air dried and then the swab inserted in transport medium and sent to laboratory.

b. For *Chlamydia*—swab from cleaned cervix; spread it on a clean special slide for immunofluorescence and put the swab in chlamydia culture medium.

c. For *Trichomonas*—put swab into the trichomonas medium (brown fluid).

d. For herpes genitalis—swab from the ulcers, spread on special slide for electron microscopy and put the swab in viral culture medium.

e. For syphilis—10 ml of clotted blood in plain container and ask for serological studies for syphilis.

Always refer the patient to the clinic for treatment, follow-up studies and contact tracing.

PSYCHOSEXUAL PROBLEMS

The most frequently occurring difficulties relate to pre-marital anxiety, frigidity, non-consumation, impotence, including premature ejaculation.

Specialized courses are available for doctors who wish to undertake further treatment in this field (*see* appendices).

FURTHER READING

Spagna V. A. and Prior R. B. (1985) *Sexually Transmitted Diseases*. New York, Marcel Dekker Inc.

Chapter 13

Abortion

INTRODUCTION

There is no true indication to admit patients to hospital who are threatening to abort (pregnancy with vaginal bleeding but no pain or cervical dilatation) and such patients should preferably be treated at home with bed rest and psychotherapy.

Similarly, patients who have had a complete abortion do not require hospital admission.

Admission to hospital is indicated for any of the other classifications of abortion.

THREATENED ABORTION

Management

Bed rest (up to shower and toilet); ultrasound examination. No drug therapy except for patients who have received progestogens in a previous successful pregnancy and who have confidence in progestogen therapy; these may receive hydroxyprogesterone caproate (*see Fig.* 13.1) which will not cause virilization of the female fetus. Psychotherapy is recommended. If ultrasound is not available human chorionic gonadotrophin assays may be used—*see Table* 13.1.

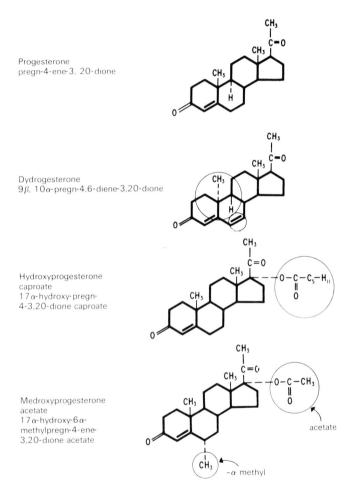

Progesterone
pregn-4-ene-3, 20-dione

Dydrogesterone
9β, 10α-pregn-4,6-diene-3,20-dione

Hydroxyprogesterone
caproate
17α-hydroxy-pregn-
4-3,20-dione caproate

Medroxyprogesterone
acetate
17α-hydroxy-6α-
methylpregn-4-ene-
3,20-dione acetate

acetate

-α methyl

Fig. 13.1. Progestogens.

INCOMPLETE ABORTION

Confirm by ultrasound. Proceed to theatre to evacuate retained products of conception. The procedure may, however, be undertaken as a ward procedure. The products should be sent for histopathology.

Ward Management of Incomplete Abortion

This method may be used for those patients who abort below 14 weeks' gestation. It may be used for abortions above 14 weeks' gestation provided that the bulk of the placenta has been passed spontaneously.

Table 13.1. Normal range human chorionic gonadotrophin titres in normal pregnancy

Days after last menstrual period	HCG (IU/l early morning urine)	
	Mean value	Range
40	8000	4000–40000
50	40000	15000–100000
60	80000	40000–200000
70 (peak)	100000	40000–400000
80	90000	40000–500000
100	70000	20000–250000
120	30000	15000–100000
140	25000	10000–50000
180	30000	10000–50000

Procedure

The patient is placed in the lithotomy position and is swabbed and draped with sterile towels. The patient is given a pre-medication of 10 mg valium and 50 mg pethidine, slowly, intravenously. This may occasionally be repeated if necessary but care must be exercised in giving these drugs to avoid overdosing the patient.

A speculum is inserted and the cervix visualized and cleansed with povidone–iodine solution. The anterior cervix is grasped with the curved single-toothed vulsellum forceps. The Karman curette equipment (*see Fig.* 13.2) is assembled and a negative pressure of approximately 635 mm is attained. (This part of the equipment is worked by the assistant nurse.)

An 8-mm Karman curette is inserted into the cervix and the vacuum is connected to the patient. The curette is gently moved up and down the uterus and is rotated through 360° until a grating feeling is observed on *all* internal surfaces of the uterus. The pressure may drop to 15 mmHg at this stage. A 6- or 10-mm Karman curette may occasionally be used. Intravenous ergometrine is not required as a routine, unless bleeding has been excessive.

Intravenous oxytocin, 10 units, may be given.

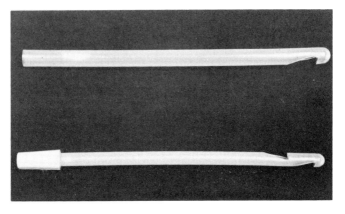

Fig. 13.2. Karman curette for first trimester termination of pregnancy.

COMPLETE ABORTION

Ultrasound examination of the uterus for confirmation. Anti-D 100 mg should be given to all rhesus negative patients having abortions (p. 158).

RECURRENT ABORTIONS

Samples of products of conception should be kept in clean, sterile containers in case chromosomal studies are requested.

Patients who habitually abort (*see* Stirratt, 1983; DeCherney and Polan, 1984) may require further investigations:

a. Electrophoresis.
b. Serum folate.
c. High vaginal swab to exclude infection (HVS).
d. Serological test for syphilis (STS).
e. X-ray chest.
f. X-ray skull for pituitary fossa when the serum prolactin is raised.
g. Mid-stream specimen of urine (MSU).
h. Blood urea.
i. Glucose tolerance test.
j. Thyroid function tests.
k. Brucella antibodies.
l. Toxoplasmosis antibodies.
m. Cytomegalovirus antibodies.
n. Cervical culture for mycoplasmas and *Chlamydia*.
o. Buccal smear—procedure (p. 121):
   i. Rinse the patient's mouth with water.
   ii. Using the rounded end of an Ayre's spatula, scrape the buccal cavity supporting the cheek with the hand.

    iii. Smear the cells and saliva along the length of a glass slide and immediately place in fixative for 10 min.

    iv. Repeat this procedure a further three times on the same area of the buccal cavity.

    v. Carry out this method on the other cheek.

    vi. There should be eight slides in all and, when fixed, should be dispatched to the cytology department.

p. Maternal karyotype.

q. Paternal karyotype.

r. Hysterosalpingogram; hysteroscopy; laparoscopy.

Treatment

Treatment is directed at the cause but if no obvious aetological factors are evident immunotherapy should be considered (Taylor and Faulk, 1981).

Pregnancy, be it on a temporary basis, is an example of successful allograph. If immune mechanisms are relevant to normal pregnancy, defects of the immune system may occasionally give rise to abnormalities of pregnancy, in particular defects of implantation and early pregnancy failure. The following immunological test systems are used to investigate possible defects of the immune mechanism in early pregnancy:

a. Typing of paternal and maternal lymphocytes for HLA antigens at the A, B, C and D loci. The purpose of this investigation is to assess the degree of genetic similarity between male and female partners as shown by the degree of HLA sharing when compared to a control group.

b. Cytotoxic testing between maternal serum and paternal lymphocytes. The purpose of this test is to assess the degree of maternal recognition of paternal antigens that the mother encounters via the fetus during pregnancy.

From the obstetric history and the immunological findings two groups can be identified.

Primary Aborters
i. No successful pregnancies by a particular partner.
ii. Sharing of more than two HLA antigens with the partner.
iii. No cytotoxic antibodies in maternal serum against paternal antigens.
Possible failed immunological recognition.

Secondary Aborters
i. One or more successful pregnancies with a particular partner OR late intra-uterine death.
ii. No abnormal HLA sharing compared to a control group.
iii. Cytotoxic antibody in maternal serum against paternal antigens.
Possible abnormal immunological recognition.

Treatment
Repeated transfusion throughout pregnancy with leucocyte encircled plasma from at least 16 different erythrocyte compatible donors.

MISSED ABORTION

If the uterus is below 12 weeks' gestation in size, a dilation and suction evacuation is appropriate. Above 12 weeks' uterine size, an intravenous infusion of prostaglandins may be elected. The dose regime is 5 μg/min of prostaglandin E_2 (PGE_2). A 5 mg ampoule of PGE_2 may be equally divided into two 500-ml bottles of 5% dextrose. This gives a concentration of 5 μg/ml. This is infused at 1 ml/min (15 drops/min). The drip may be increased gradually up to 60 drops/min if no response occurs. Alternatively extra-amniotic prostaglandins may be used and are recommended (p. 137). The possibility of disseminated intra-vascular coagulopathy should be remembered.

THERAPEUTIC ABORTION

The resident should confirm that the necessary forms are completed:

a. Certificate A (green form).
b. Certificate HSA4 (buff form).
c. Contraceptive advice should be given. This is normally arranged at the gynaecology clinic but, if required, may be via a family planning clinic (FPA) on a local basis. Otherwise the patients or their GPs will make the necessary FPA appointment. Anti-D 100 mg should be given to all rhesus negative patients.

First Trimester Abortion

Vacuum termination of pregnancies (*see* p. 131).

Second Trimester Abortion

The extra-ovular routine is recommended as it is the simplest to use and it is associated with fewer side-effects. Patients should preferably be admitted for prostaglandin termination one day prior to routine lists so that any required evacuation could be placed on the appropriate routine list.

Preparation of the Patient

In the dorsal or lithotomy position, the vulva is cleansed with Hibitane. A bivalve speculum is inserted and the cervix visualized and cleansed with povidone–iodine solution. A size 14 Foley catheter is inserted through the cervix using sponge holding forceps and the balloon filled with 30–40 ml sterile water.

Occasionally the cervix may need to be controlled using a single toothed tenaculum. The catheter is spigotted, the speculum removed and the patient returns to her bed and is connected via manometer tubing to the prostaglandin/oxytocin solution on the Sage pump. The danger of potential water intoxication should be remembered.

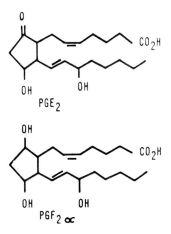

Fig. 3.3. Prostaglandins.

Solution

Five mg prostaglandin E_2 4 ml are injected down the manometer tube and catheter to fill these tubes and to give a 2 ml bolus to the patient. Thereafter the solution is infused at 3·5–4 ml/min until abortion occurs. Following the abortion a curettage is usually required. This may be done as a ward procedure using the portable Karman curette equipment.

SEPTIC ABORTION

Blood cultures should be requested. Septic shock, its diagnosis and management should be considered. Antibodies should be prescribed prior to curettage.

Brief Blood Culture Instructions

These should be discussed with the technician on call outside working hours (*see* p. 166).

At the Bedside

Careful asepsis. Record the brief clinical and antibiotic history on the request card (the laboratory will add penicillinase if necessary). Instant incubation is required.

Normal Investigations

Three venepunctures (separated by convenient but not excessive time) each of 10 ml should be taken and divided equally between two identical bottles. Record time on bottle label so that the laboratory knows which pair is which.

Acute Infections

Two venepunctures (separated by the shortest of intervals) each of 10 ml should be taken and divided equally between two identical bottles. Record time on bottle label so that the laboratory knows which pair is which.

HYDATIDIFORM MOLE (p. 180)

The diagnosis is made by ultrasonography based on clinical suspicion (large- or small-for-date uterus; general malaise). The uterus is emptied using vacuum curettage or prostaglandins but two units of blood should be available in the event of a haemorrhage. A repeat curettage is undertaken after one month and the patient referred to the Regional Endocrine Investigation Centre for review and monitoring (*see* Appendix II).

ECTOPIC PREGNANCY

The possibility of ectopic pregnancy should always be considered; clinically it may present as pelvic inflammatory disease (p. 167). If in doubt admit the patient to hospital for diagnostic laparoscopy.

FURTHER READING

DeCherney A. and Polan M. L. (1984) Evaluation and management of habitual abortion. *Br. J. Hosp. Med.* 261–268

Leading Article (1983) Maternal blocking antibodies, the fetal allograph and recurrent abortion. *Lancet* **ii**, 1175–1176

Stirratt G. (1983) Recurrent abortion—a review. *Br. J. Obstet. Gynaecol.* **90**, 881–883

Taylor C. and Faulk W. P. (1981) Prevention of recurrent abortion with leucocyte transfusion. *Lancet* **ii**, 68

Chapter 14

Infertility

INTRODUCTION

Separate clinics for patients suffering from infertility have been advocated, where both partners may be counselled. A full history from both partners is required, initial investigations instigated and appropriate treatment advised.

Most infertility investigations can be undertaken on an outpatient basis by the general practitioner and hospital admission only recommended for laparoscopic assessment of the pelvic organs.

INVESTIGATIONS COMMONLY UTILIZED

Patients should always be tested for rubella immunity prior to treatment. Investigations include:

Semen analysis
Postcoital test
Hysterosalpingography
Laparoscopy and hydrotubation
Endocrinological investigations:
　　LH
　　FSH
　　Prolactin
　　Progesterone
　　Thyroid studies
　　Cortisol
　　24-hour urine oestrogen

X-ray of pituitary fossa
Chromosomal studies
Basal body temperature
Cervical mucus.

FACTORS INVOLVED

The appropriate management for the different factors is
given below.

Male Factors
See Table 14.1 for normal semen analysis.

Table 14.1. Normal semen analysis

Semen count	> 20 million/ml
Progressive motility	$> 60\%$
Morphology	$< 40\%$ abnormal head forms

Azoospermia
If confirmed on three semen analyses, advise adoption or
artificial insemination using donor semen (Ledward, 1983).

Oligospermia
FSH level; karyotype; ligation of variocele; mid-cycle
coitus; hypothermia to testes.

Sexual Disorders
Refer to psychosexual clinic.

Female Factors

Anovulation

Ovulation stimulation with clomiphene citrate, bromocriptine, gonadotrophins, LHRH or FSH.

Tubal Factors

Microsurgical techniques; *in vitro* fertilization.

Uterine Factors

Myomectomy for leiofibromata.

Cervical Factors

Postcoital testing for confirmation of cervical hostility.

Vaginal Factors

Correct infection, consider referral to psychosexual clinic.

OVULATION INDUCTION

Investigations

Evidence of Tubal Patency

This is obtained by either salpingography or dye insufflation. Together with evidence of male fertility, it should be confirmed before treatment.

Non-ovulation and Oligomenorrhoea

Investigation of non-ovulation and oligomenorrhoea involves the following (*see* p. 120):

a. Plasma LH and/or FSH: high levels indicate exogenous gonadotrophins and are unlikely to be of any use.

b. Serum prolactin.
c. Skull X-ray: if oligomenorrhoea or secondary amenorrhoea or serum prolactin elevated.
d. Plasma thyroxine and T_3 uptake.
e. Plasma cortisol: at 11:00 hours.
f. 24-hour oestrogens and preganediol as a baseline pre-treatment level.

Exclusion of Local Factors

High vaginal swab and smear; dilatation and curettage (D & C); histopathology and endometrial culture for exclusion of tuberculosis.

Temperature Charts

Temperature charts should be started at the time of initiation of therapy.

Treatment (Ledward, 1984)

Bromocriptine

Bromocriptine therapy if the serum prolactin is raised (normal assay levels may differ between varying laboratories).

Combined Therapy with Clomiphene Citrate and HCG

All patients should be tried on this regime before proceeding to gonadotrophin (pergonal) therapy.

The following regime is suggested:

Day 4 of cycle: 24-hour urine collection for baseline oestrogen levels.

Day 5–Day 9: 50 mg clomiphene/day, increasing to 150 mg daily if there has been no previous evidence of success with clomiphene citrate.

Day 10–Day 11: 24-hour urine sample—for total oestrogen levels. (Clomiphene citrate may be prescribed in low doses without oestrogen monitoring initially.)

Day 14: If total oestrogen levels fall between 31 and 125 μg/24 h, ovulation should be triggered with HCG 3000–6000 IU.

Day 24: A further 24-hour urine collection should be obtained for total oestrogens and blood for serum progesterone.

Gonadotrophin Therapy

AMENORRHOEIC PATIENTS Patients should be encouraged to achieve their normal weight (*Table* 1.1) prior to treatment.

Admit the patient for the initial month of therapy, thereafter outpatient monitoring is acceptable.

a. The object of pergonal therapy is to promote follicular maturation to the stage where, by stimulating the normal mid-cycle luteinizing hormone (LH) surge, the addition of human chorionic gonadotrophin (HCG) will induce ovulation and the formation of a corpus luteum.

b Pergonal regime (human menopausal gonadotrophin):

Day 1: Collect 24-hour sample of urine, measure total volume; pelvic examination.

Day 2: Give 5 ampoules of pergonal after 24 hours (5 × 75 l/U).

Day 3: No treatment.

Day 4: Repeat Day 2; start collection of 24-hour urine collection.

Day 5: Repeat Day 1.

Day 6: Repeat Day 4.

Day 7: Repeat Day 1.

Day 8: No treatment.

Day 9: Give 10 000 IU HCG if oestrogen response is satisfactory.

When to give HCG:

180 nmol/24 h (50 mg/24 h) of total urinary oestrogen = follicular development inadequate; no HCG. 514 nmol/24 h (140 mg/24 h) of total urinary oestrogen = increased risk of ovarian hyperstimulation; no HCG.

Monitor ovarian stimulation by ultrasonography.

If result is between 180–514 nmol/24 h give HCG.

Patients should be advised to have *intercourse* on the day preceding, and the two days following the HCG injection.

c. Classification of patients: Experience has shown gonadotrophin therapy (pergonal) to be particularly effective in two main groups of anovulatory infertile women, as shown in *Table* 14.2.

d. Precautions:

    i. Pergonal therapy is abandoned when an effective response cannot be obtained.

    ii. Certain pathological conditions should be excluded or treated before commencing gonadotrophin therapy. Patients selected should meet the following criteria:

        Positive indication, i.e. they should wish to become pregnant.

        Fertile or potentially fertile partner.

        Potentially responsive ovaries, i.e. ovarian dysgenesis or early menopause should be excluded.

        Reproductive organs compatible with fertility—normal vagina and uterus, patent fallopian tubes.

        No evidence of untreated endocrine disorders such as hyperprolactinaemia, hypothyroidism or adrenocortical deficiency which may lead to anovulation.

        No evidence of untreated pituitary tumours.

No untreated organic causes for abnormal bleeding patterns.

iii. All patients should be examined vaginally before embarking on subsequent course of injections.

e. Liaison with pathology laboratory:

i. The pathology laboratory would like to be notified by the prescriber *24 hours in advance* of any course of treatment. This enables them to spot the bottles as soon as they appear and thus minimize delay.

Table 14.2. Classification of patients

Group 1*	Group 2†
Primary or secondary amenorrhoea, including patient with hypo-gonadotrophic ovarian failure, complete or partial hypopituitarism, or hypothalamic–pituitary failure	Menstrual cycle disturbances including amenorrhoea
Low endogenous oestrogen activity; urinary oestrogens < 37 nmol/24 h (< 10 μg/24 h) or plasma oestrogens < 370 pmol/l (< 100 pg/ml)	Distinct endogenous oestrogen activity; urinary oestrogens > 37 nmol/24 h (> 10 μg/24 h) or plasma oestrogens > 370 pmol/l (> 100 pg/ml)
Endogenous gonadotrophins low or unmeasurable	Endogenous gonadotrophins in normal range or fluctuating
Normal plasma prolactin levels	Normal plasma prolactin levels
Failure to bleed after progestogen challenge	Menstrual bleed after progestogen challenge
No detectable pituitary tumour	

From the World Health Organisation Scientific Group (*WHO Technical Report Series*, 1973), with modifications proposed by the WHO Scientific Group Meeting (Hamburg, 1976).

* Pergonal is the treatment of choice for patients in Group 1.
† For patients in Group 2; drugs stimulating endogenous gonadotrophin release, e.g. clomiphene, are generally recommended as first-line treatment. Patients who do not respond to repeated courses of such agents should be considered for treatment with pergonal.

ii. Patients should be asked to report personally to the pathology laboratory when they take their first sample. Patients will then be shown the most convenient place to leave the samples.

iii. Because of the difficulties at the weekends, treatment is best started on Wednesday or Thursday. Patients should start their 24-hour base level collections on Tuesday or Wednesday.

MENSTRUATING PATIENTS The same directions as above apply with the following additions:

a. Injections should start on the third day of bleeding and at the latest Day 5.

b. Initial injections should be 1 ampoule (75 IU)—this dose should be doubled by Day 7 if response is inadequate.

Pergonal therapy may be monitored using the free services provided by Serono Laboratories UK Ltd.

Luteinizing Hormone Releasing Hormone

Pulsatile administration of LHRH delivered via specially designed miniaturized pumps that inject 15 μg of LHRH at 90-min intervals has been successful in inducing ovulation for patients with hypogonadotrophic hypogonadism and megalocystic ovarian syndrome (*see* Vickery and Nestor, 1984; Mason, 1984).

UROFOLLITROPHIN This is a preparation of gonadotrophin extracted from human menopausal urine. It possesses follicle stimulating hormone activity but no luteinizing hormone activity. It is indicated for the subfertile patient with polycystic ovarian disease–anovulatory infertility, menstrual disturbances, hirsutism, acne, obesity, bilateral polycystic ovaries and a raised luteinizing hormone (LH):

follicle stimulating hormone (FSH) ratio of more than 3:1. Urofollitrophin is indicated for patients who have failed to respond to clomiphene citrate (*see* Stein and Leventhal, 1935; Katz, 1981).

SUMMARY

Infertility is a distressing symptom. It is only possible to achieve the best possible fertility status for each individual couple, but a successful pregnancy is not always possible. *In vitro* fertilization may be necessary in cases of 'idiopathic infertility' (Warnock, 1984).

Support and explanation of the situation is important, but the psychology of infertility remains complex with some patients only wishing to negate their barren status without the positive end result of a healthy child.

FURTHER READING

Katz M. (1981) Polycystic ovaries. *Clin. Obstet. Gynaecol.* **8**, 715–731

Ledward R. S. (1983) Social and biological factors as determinants of success rates in donor insemination. DM Thesis, University of Nottingham

Ledward R. S. (1984) *Drug Treatment in Gynaecology.* London, Butterworths

Mason P., Adams J. Morris D. V. *et al.* (1984) Induction of ovulation with pulsatile luteinizing hormone releasing hormone. *Br. Med. J.* **288**, 181–185

Stein I. F. and Leventhal M. L. (1935) Amenorrhoea associated with bilateral polycystic ovaries. *Am. J. Obstet. Gynecol.* **29**, 181–191

Vickery B. H. and Nestor J. J. (1984) *LHRH and its Analogs: Contraceptive and Therapeutic Applications.* Lancaster, MTP

Warnock M. (1984) *Report on the Committee of Inquiry into Human Fertilization and Embryology.* Cmnd. Cl 314, London, HMSO

Chapter 15

Cytology, Colposcopy, Histopathology

INTRODUCTION

Liaison with heads of other departments is strongly recommended. The RMO should become efficient in routine colposcopy and the diagnosis and management of positive cervical smears.

PAPANICOLAOU'S SMEAR

The resident should ensure he understands the indications for taking a cervical smear and, if in doubt as to the correct procedure, receives instruction from his senior colleagues. An Ayre spatula or cervical swab may be used and the squamocolumnar junction should be scraped. The smear should be placed on a glass slide and fixed immediately.

Indications for cervical smears include:

a. Antenatal booking clinics.
b. Postnatal clinic visit.
c. Routine gynaecological assessment in hospital.
d. Annual routine smears in sexually active women.
e. If in doubt when last performed.

The smear should be fixed and the cervical smear request form fully completed, ensuring that the following are recorded:

a. Previous cytology reference numbers.
b. Relevant previous history, e.g. previous positive smears or cone biopsy, hormone therapy and date of last menstrual period.
c. Clear identification of source and name of consultant and general practitioner.

Smear results should be signed by the registrar prior to filing the notes.

COLPOSCOPY

All patients who have a Grade 3 or 4 (DHSS classification) smear should be referred for colposcopy (*see* Singer, 1977).

The colposcopist must have had adequate training and experience to recognize and biopsy the changes associated with cervical intra-epithelial neoplasia (CIN), micro-invasion and frank carcinoma. Ultimately the decision on treatment is made by the consultant with reference to the colposcopy findings and the histology.

Apparatus for Colposcopy

Apparatus required for a colposcopy includes:

a. A colposcope with a magnification of × 8.
b. Cusco speculum.
c. Sponge-holding forceps.
d. Sharp biopsy forceps with a *small* head.
e. Normal saline and 3% acetic acid in separate bottles.
f. Cotton wool balls.
g. Cotton buds on a long stick ('Q' tips) to clean the cervix.
h. A comfortable couch for the patient to lie in a modified lithotomy position.
i. Colposcopist's chair.

COLPOSCOPY CLINIC

1-2 NAME ______ 5 AGE ______ 3 STATUS ______ UNIT No. ______

DATE ______ H.M.O. ______ REFERRING DR. ______

8	9	9	9	9
Attending for cancer detection:	Pre menopausal.	Post menopausal.	Nullipera.	Para.
	12	11	10	1–9

MACROSCOPIC FINDINGS: (Cervix)	NORMAL	NOT SUSPICIOUS OF CARCINOMA	SUSPICIOUS OF CARCINOMA	OBVIOUS CARCINOMA
	1	2	3	4

11
COLPOSCOPIC FINDINGS:
(Cervix)

After Iodine – 12

All Iodine positive	1
Iodine negative	2
Sharp	3
Intermediate	4
Parakeratosis 5	+ 6, + 7, + 8

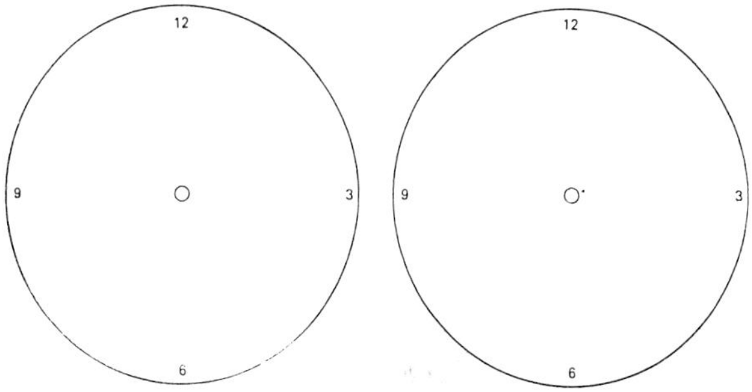

UNSATISFACTORY:	NORMAL:	NOT SUSPICIOUS: of Carcinoma	ATYPICAL:	SUSPICIOUS: of Carcinoma	OBVIOUS: Carcinoma
0	1	2	3	4	5

Comment:– ______

BIOPSY: Not recommended: 6 Recommended – IN CLINIC 7 IN HOSPITAL 8

30
CYTOLOGY: Result: NEGATIVE: 1 SUSPICIOUS: 2 POSITIVE: 3

WHTSO

Fig. 15.1. Colposcopy report form.

Treatment for CIN

Treatment for CIN includes:

a. Laser therapy if the upper limit of the lesion in the endocervix can be seen.
b. Cone biopsy if the upper limit cannot be seen or if micro-invasion is suspected.
c. Diathermy under colposcopic control under general anaesthesia.
d. 'Cold' coagulation (Duncan, 1983).
e. Cryocautery in some suitable cases.

Follow-up

After treatment the patient should be recolposcoped and the smear repeated in 3–4 months' time.

If normal, smears should be repeated twice six-monthly and then annually.

HISTOPATHOLOGY

Histology Request Cards

These must always record the following in addition to clear patient identification and brief clinical information:

a. Date of last menstrual period.
b. Hormone therapy including oral contraception.
c. Previous histology reference numbers where relevant.
d. Relevant cytology reference numbers.
e. Name of consultant.
f. Name of ward.

Placental Histology

Histological examination of most placentas is completely unrewarding and wasteful of skill and resources. Placentas should only be submitted for pathological examination if it is likely that it can contribute positive information. Placentas with small areas of infarction and slightly gritty surfaces in patients with normal deliveries and antenatal examinations are a particularly unnecessary burden to the department. Placental histological examination should largely be restricted to abnormalities identified on gross inspection of the placenta after delivery and in the case of:

a. When deficient placental formation is identified prior to delivery.
b. When systemic diseases implicate the pregnancy.
c. When serious congenital abnormalities are identified in the newborn stillbirths.

Gynaecological Specimens

See p. 194.

FURTHER READING

Duncan I. (1983) The semen cold coagulator in the management of cervical intraepithelial neoplasia. *Clin. Obstet. Gynaecol.* **26**, 996–1006

Singer A. (1977) Cancer of the cervix. *Hospital Update*, 555–565

Chapter 16

Haematology

BLOOD TRANSFUSION

All patients on whom surgery is contemplated must have their blood group determined at the earliest possible opportunity (usually the first outpatient consultation). The transfusion laboratory will then be able to inform the gynaecologist that additional notice will be required for provision of blood if the patient has one of the less common blood groups.

Blood Grouping and Cross-matching (suggested procedures)

Blood Grouping

All expectant mothers will have their ABO and rhesus group determined at booking and further samples will be required later in pregnancy from those women who are rhesus negative.

Cross-matching

Blood of all groups is usually in short supply and should be used as economically as possible. Remember also, blood transfusion carries potential risks for the patient; do not transfuse without adequate clinical indication.

A request for grouping/cross-matching must be made on the appropriate transfusion form and it is important that all the information asked for is given. At least 24 hours' notice for requests for blood for transfusion and at least 48 hours' notice if six or more units of blood are required.

Emergency requests will be dealt with at all times, but it takes *two hours* to cross-match blood safely; any shorter period increases the risk of inadequately cross-matched blood.

Cross-matched blood will be kept for 24 hours from the time for which it was requested. It will then be automatically withdrawn unless the laboratory is requested to retain it.

If the patient has received a blood transfusion more than 48 hours previously, another serum sample is required. Special care should be taken when blood is taken for cross-matching and this task should not be delegated to the nursing staff.

The bottle itself should be completed with the patient's surname, Christian name, date of birth, address and signed by the doctor actually taking the blood. This is important as the blood is labelled according to the details on the blood samples rather than against the date expressed on the blood transfusion request form, as sometimes these disagree. It cannot be emphasized too strongly that the data on the blood sample bottle be completed at the bedside.

If difficulty in providing blood is anticipated due to the possession of an uncommon blood group or the presence of an irregular antibody, the consultant obstetrician will be informed by the blood transfusion service. It is then the responsibility of the obstetrician to inform the transfusion laboratory that blood will be required to stand by for delivery or operation; 48 hours' notice should be provided for elective lower segment caesarean section.

Blood is an expensive and potentially dangerous product.

It should be available for potential use but held in reserve in the majority of cases. The transfer of potential infection has been recently highlighted by the publicity relating to possible transmission of the acquired immune deficiency syndrome (AIDS).

Serum Hepatitis (Safety Precautions Against)

You are responsible for marking 'special risk' patients on the request forms. Laboratory staff collecting and handling blood samples are dependent on this information for alerting them to take special precautions to avoid infection:

a. Gloves should be worn whilst taking the patient's blood.
b. The blood sample must be sent to the laboratory in a plastic bag.
c. The pathology request form should not be placed inside the plastic bag.
d. Both the pathology form and the outside of the plastic bag should be labelled with a 'Hepatitis risk' sticker.

Possible Transmission of the Acquired Immune Deficiency Syndrome to Hospital Personnel

It has become apparent that the blood of certain groups of patients may be particularly likely to contain HTLV-III, the causative agent of AIDS. Recent evidence suggests that hospital personnel may acquire the virus, if they sustain needle stick injuries whilst handling HTLV-III infected blood.

It is therefore recommended that the blood of: (a) patients with haemophilia, (b) homosexuals, and (c) intravenous drug abuses should be treated in the same way as if it were hepatitis B positive.

OTHER BLOOD PRODUCTS

Other blood products such as platelets, fresh frozen plasma and human plasma protein fraction are available for certain haematology problems. Discuss any blood product requirements with the junior medical staff in haematology.

If blood products are considered necessary in addition to solutions such as low-molecular-weight dextrans for blood volume replacement, then the product of choice is human plasma protein fraction. Supplies of this material may be limited, in which case dried human plasma will be issued instead.

Fibrinogen is available from the transfusion laboratory for cases in which fibrinogen deficiency has been demonstrated. Fresh frozen plasma and platelet concentrates may be indicated and discussion with the haematologist on call is advised. In order that these blood products should be readily available, it is necessary for users to appreciate that they will have to accept an increasing number of units of red cells from which the plasma has been removed.

ANTICOAGULANT CONTROL (Suggested procedure)

Anticoagulant therapy in gynaecological and postpartum patients should be along the lines indicated by the anticoagulant chart and the information provided below. The following regime is recommended for starting patients on anticoagulants. Warfarin sodium is the drug of first choice (with or without immediate heparinization). A single large

Table 16.1

Age (years)	First day	Second day	Third day
Under 50	30 mg	*Give no warfarin*	Laboratory staff will do thrombosis test; give no warfarin until recommended dose has been decided by haematologist
50–70	30 mg		
Over 70	15–21 mg		

Send anticoagulant card to haematology laboratory requesting anticoagulant dosage control and stating date of initial dose.

dose is given initially, the size of which varies with age, body weight, degree of illness. In general, old or very ill or very small people require smaller initial doses; younger, heavier or relatively fit people should have higher initial doses. The recommended doses are average and should be adjusted in accordance with the considerations shown in *Table* 16.1.

When a patient is to be discharged on anticoagulant treatment notify the haematology laboratory in good time by sending the anticoagulant card with the section headed 'Request for Outpatient Control' completed.

PREVENTION OF RHESUS HAEMOLYTIC DISEASE OF THE NEWBORN

All rhesus negative women without anti-D in their serum must receive anti-D immunoglobulin when undergoing:

a. Delivery of a rhesus positive infant.

b. Termination of pregnancy (by any means).

c. Spontaneous abortion.

d. External cephalic version.

e. Amniocentesis (for whatever reason).

Anti-D should be given *within 24 hours* if possible, and within 72 hours at the very latest.

FURTHER READING

Letsky E. A. (Ed.) (1985) Coagulation problems in obstetrics during pregnancy. In *Current Reviews in Obstetrics and Gynaecology*, Vol. 10. Edinburgh, Churchill Livingstone

Chapter 17

Clinical Chemistry

INTRODUCTION

Residents should make early liaison with laboratory staff and discuss specific problems with them.

ROUTINE BLOOD CHEMISTRY

Sample requirements for all blood tests: 5 ml blood in an orange tube.

The principal exceptions are:

Endocrinology
Proteins　　　　　　　} 5 ml in a plain white tube
Glycosylated haemoglobin

Key Reference Ranges (Adult) for Blood Chemistry

Sodium	127–145 mmol/l
Potassium	3·5–5·0 mmol/l
Calcium	2·1–2·6 mmol/l
Bicarbonate	24–30 mmol/l
Urea*	2·5–6·6 mmol/l
Creatinine*	80–180 mmol/l
Alkaline phosphatase†	75–245 IU/l
Aspartate aminotransferase (AST)	13–38 IU/l

Total bilirubin   7–20 μmol/l
γ-Glutamyltranspeptidase (γ-Gt)
    of liver function female   7–32 mol/l

* Decreased levels found in normal pregnancy.
† Levels increased in pregnancy from placenta.

Electrophoresis of alkaline phosphatase iso-enzymes is available to distinguish between increase from liver, intestinal or placental origin where there is clinical doubt.

ENDOCRINE TESTS

Thyroid Function Testing

The laboratory assessment of thyroid function is expensive and, as thyroid function tests are often asked for inappropriately or indiscriminately, the following guidelines are made available:

a. T_4 should be requested for preliminary investigation of thyroid dysfunction and to monitor treated thyrotoxics.
b. TSH should be requested for monitoring patients receiving thyroxine for primary hypothyroidism, to ensure that therapy is adequate.

The laboratory will initiate further tests where the initial result does not provide adequate information for proper interpretation, thus:

a. T_3 will be measured where the T_4 is raised or high–normal and there are clinical indications of thyrotoxicosis.
b. TS_4 will be measured where the T_4 is low or low–normal and potential hypothyroidism is being investigated.

Full clinical and therapy details must be provided in order that the most appropriate tests are carried out.

Where other tests are specifically requested, the information supplied must indicate the reasons for this, for example, to identify overtreatment, or when there is TSH deficiency, in a patient receiving thyroxine (a total T_3 measurement is probably of more use in these situations than a T_4 measurement).

Where total hormone level results do not appear to fit the clinical picture, further testing may be useful and the laboratory should be contacted. Free T_3 and T_4 measurements may provide more useful information in certain groups of patients, e.g. borderline and treated thyrotoxics. At present the T_3 uptake test, to obtain a free thyroxine index can be measured where there is an indication that the total binding globulin (TBG) may be altered, e.g. in women on the Pill or pregnant.

Please note that total T_3 levels are not considered useful in investigating hypothyroidism and TSH assays are insufficiently sensitive to distinguish a normal from a suppressed level in thyrotoxicosis (a more sensitive TSH assay is being sought).

Normal Range of Thyroid Function Tests

Oestrogen therapy in late pregnancy can affect thyroid function test results.

T_4	55–155 mmol/l
TSH	< 5·5 mU/l
T_3	0·80–2·46 mmol/l

The free thyroxine index is the most reliable measure of thyroid function and is unaffected by pregnancy or oral contraceptives.

Feto-placental Function Assessment (Serum Oestriol)

Sample: 5 ml clotted blood (white tube).

The test results are only useful if available as a series. However, the test is extremely expensive and should only be requested when clinical management will be determined by the results.

As with α-fetoprotein results, the interpretation of oestriol results is dependent upon accurate knowledge of the gestational age. Ensure that request forms indicate the gestational age.

Measurement of human placental lactogen is also possible, but has to be carried out at one of the national supraregional assay service laboratories. Please make arrangements with the laboratory before collecting the sample.

Endocrine Investigation of Infertility

The endocrinological investigation of infertility, should only be considered after exclusion of all other causes in either partner. If endocrine investigations are embarked upon, a logical structured protocol must be followed—the laboratory can give guidance.

Sample collection and particularly result interpretation in females must be related to the menstrual cycle history, e.g. progesterone studies virtually always require sample collection on Day 21. The request form must give full clinical details.

A single result or investigation is of limited value. To assist in the interpretation of results, some key reference ranges are listed below:

FSH	Follicular and luteal phases	0·5–5 U/l
	Ovulatory peak	>2 times baseline
LH	Follicular and luteal phases	3–12 U/l
	Ovulatory peak	>3 times baseline
Progesterone	Mid-luteal peak (Day 21)	>30 nmol/l
	Non-secretory	<4 nmol/l

Oestradiol	Early follicular	74–868 pmol/l
	Luteal	368–1100 pmol/l
	Mid-cycle	735–1840 pmol/l
	Post-menopausal	< 184 pmol/l
Prolactin		Up to 400 mU/l
Testosterone		9–24 nmol/l (♂)
		0·5–2·5 nmol/l (♀)
Thyroxine (T$_4$)		55–155 nmol/l
Tri-iodothyronine (T$_3$)		0·8–2·5 nmol/l
TSH		0·08–7·5 mU/l

NB The reference ranges above are for guidance only: some of the assays may have to be carried out in laboratories using methods with ranges different to those quoted above.

SPECIAL TESTS

Amniocentesis

a. For rhesus disease   5 ml in dark bottle.
b. For α-fetoprotein   5 ml in dark bottle.
c. For karyotyping   5 ml in dark bottle.

Glucose Tolerance Test

a. Short test (adequate for most cases), 2 ml fluoride bottle.

Fast from previous night, no breakfast, no tobacco. Take a fasting blood glucose specimen. Give 50 g glucose or 235 ml 'Lucozade' or according to body weight and take a further sample at 2 hours.

b. Full test (lag storage curve, renal threshold study etc.). Preparation as above. Test as above with additional blood specimens at 0·5, 1 and 1·5 hours and urine specimens fasting and at 1 and 2 hours.

Renal Function

a. Creatinine clearance test: An accurate 24-hour urine save plus a 5 ml blood specimen taken during the save

b. Osmolality of serum and urine Serum-clotted blood
Urine-casual specimen

c. Serum and urinary electrolytes and urea Blood

Useful in management of advanced renal failure or acute situations Urine must be full 24-hour sample

d. Catecholamines 24-hour urine save with 15 ml concentrated hydrochloric acid (*danger*)

Preliminary dieting no longer required

Methyldopa is unlikely to interfere, but give details of any antihypertensive therapy on the request card

Maternal Serum α-Fetoprotein

Maternal serum α-fetoprotein measurements as a screening test for fetal open neural defects can only be meaningfully carried out between the sixteenth and nineteenth weeks of gestation. Moreover, as the interpretation of the results is critically dependent upon an exact knowledge of gestational age, ultrasound scanning should be carried out at the time of the blood test.

Sample: 5 ml clotted blood (white tube).

Interpretation: 80% of open neural tube defects will have an α-fetoprotein result greater than 2·5 times the median value for that gestational age. Falsely high results may be obtained if it is a multiple pregnancy, if there is threatened miscarriage, and some congenital malformations.

Chapter 18

Microbiology

INTRODUCTION

Early liaison with the microbiology department is most important. The department should always be contacted where there is doubt regarding diagnostic or therapeutic dilemmas.

COLLECTION OF SPECIMENS

Specimens for microbiology include:

Mid-stream specimen of urine.
High vaginal and cervical swabs.
Pus from abdominal wounds.
Fluid collected from pouch of Douglas by laparoscopy or culdoscopy.

Mid-stream Specimen of Urine

An antibiotic may be selected pending sensitivities of any organism. Urines should be collected in special borate bottles which stabilize the bacterial count overnight.

Vaginal/Cervical Swabs

A transport medium, black and semi-solid, is used when *Candida* on gonococci are suspected and for general microbiology. When *Trichomonas vaginalis* is suspected the trichomonas medium (brown and fluid) is used.

165

Specimens for Gram-positive staining are sent with no medium. Pus should be collected into a dry, sterile container rather than a swab taken from pus. If swabs are necessary, transport media should be used.

Diagnosis of Wound Infection

This is a clinical bedside diagnosis which may not require antibiotic therapy. The laboratory may be able to help with the recognition of the causative organism. The isolation of an organism, however, does not mean that there is infection; colonizing and commensal organisms are universal. If a generalized infection or septicaemia is suspected, *blood cultures* should be taken.

BLOOD CULTURES

Brief Blood Culture Instructions

At the Bedside

Careful asepsis. Record the brief clinical and antibiotic history on the request card. (The laboratory will add penicillinase if necessary.) Instant incubation is required. Blood culture bottles contain a small amount of H particle which allows for the rapid detection of bacterial growth. The radioactivity is only a hazard if a bottle is broken.

NORMAL INVESTIGATION Three venepunctures (separated by convenient but not large time intervals) each of 10 ml should be taken and divided equally between two identical bottles. Record time on bottle labels so that the laboratory knows which pair is which.

ACUTE INFECTIONS Two venepunctures (separated by the shortest of intervals) each of 10 ml should be taken and divided equally between two identical bottles. Record time on bottle labels so that the laboratory knows which pair is which.

PELVIC INFLAMMATORY DISEASE

Ectopic pregnancy should always be considered in the differential diagnosis.

Routine Investigations

These should include:

Haemoglobin.
Full blood count and differential, white cell count.
Sedimentation rate.
Mid-stream specimen of urine.
Cervical swab.
Cervical smear.

Other Procedures

Other procedures to be considered include:

Chlamydia fluorescein antibody tests.
Ultrasonography for pregnancy.
Blood culture.
Laparoscopy.
Referral to a clinic for sexually transmitted diseases.

Treatment (p. 169)

PROPHYLAXIS (p. 190)

Prophylactic antibiotics, including metronidazole, may be used in gynaecological surgery; long-acting sulphonamides may be given prior to catheterization, but many urinary tract organisms are now resistant to sulphonamides (Hawkins, 1983; Stirrat and Beeley, 1986).

ANTIBIOTIC OF CHOICE

The antibiotic of choice is the one to which the organism is sensitive and which is not harmful to the mother and possible fetus.

Remember, mothers and babies are particularly prone to infection and maternity units are one of the departments where *cross infection* occurs. *Always collect samples before treating.* Many organisms are becoming resistant; seek advice if there is not a therapeutic response in 48 hours. Certain antibiotics are contraindicated in pregnancy and lactation. (*See* Zuspan and Christian, 1983.)

Specific Infected Sites

Abdominal Wound Infections

Deep sepsis is not uncommon after caesarean section.

Cause is usually *Staphylococcus aureus* and/or anaerobes.

Treatment is flucloxacillin and metronidazole *or* augmentin *or* erythromycin and metronidazole.

Vaginal Wounds

These include episiotomies, perineal abscesses, puerperal infections.

Cause is usually anaerobic, occasionally staphylococcal or streptococcal.

Treatment is as for wounds.

Breast Abscesses

Cause is usually *Staphylococcus aureus,* sometimes anaerobic streptococci.

Treatment is flucloxacillin (or fucidic acid).

Vaginal Infections and Pelvic Inflammatory Disease

Common causes are *Candida*, *Trichomonas*, anaerobic vaginosis (*Gardnerella*).

Treatment is metronidazole and antifungals.

Less common causes are *Chlamydia*, herpes simplex, gonococcal infections. Most of these are sexually transmitted; remember to ask about partner.

Treatment is erythromycin, acyclovir, penicillin (but take consultant's or medical microbiologist's advice before treating).

Pelvic Inflammatory Disease (p. 167)

Most of the above organisms can cause pelvic inflammatory disease (PID). Collect samples if possible.

Treatment—augmentin plus erythromycin covers most of the causes.

Urinary Tract Infection

a. Cystitis is very common and when recurrent a gynaecological problem is often the cause; upper tract problems are rare causes.

Catheterization will often introduce infection. Short-term indwelling catheters should be sampled twice a week (Mondays and Thursdays). Long-term indwelling catheters will always be infected. Only treat before a surgical procedure or if the patient has general symptoms. Only neurogenic bladders are associated with upper urinary tract infection.

b. Acute, recurrent and chronic pyelonephritis though less common are much more serious and likely to be associated with renal tract abnormalities. A full urology 'work-up' should be considered in these cases.

c. Pyelonephritis of pregnancy can usually be prevented by screening in early pregnancy and treating asymptomatic bacteriuria. Treatment involves a short course (3 days) of one of the following:

Try first: trimethoprim, nitrofurantoin, nalidixic acid. If intolerant, cefaclor.

Use ampicillin *only* if laboratory report indicates organism sensitive.

Reserve augmentin for difficult cases (*see below*).

d. Upper severe pyelonephritis—collect blood culture as well as urine before treatment: This can be very serious, do not waste time with oral agents.

Use cefotaxime i.v. 2 g, 8-hourly; halve dose when there is a therapeutic response. Change to oral agents when recovered according to sensitivities.

Add gentamicin if no clinical response or change to piperacillin if not responding.

e. Less severe pyelonephritis e.g. slight temperature and loin tenderness: use augmentin.

Chest Infection

Most commonly postsurgical bronchitis but can be serious. Collect sputum if possible. Treat with Amoxycillin.

Exclude pneumonia on X-ray. Remember influenza can lead to life-threatening bronchopneumonia even in young women.

Prophylaxis for Cardiac Cases

Available regimens include:

Gentamicin i.v. + ampicillin i.v.—
    1 g 30 min before procedure.
    1·5 mg/kg + metronidazole i.v. or suppositories.
Erythromycin 500 mg (lactobionate) if penicillin allergic.
Repeat dose twice.

GENTAMICIN AND GENTAMICIN BLOOD LEVELS

Indications

Gentamicin used alone is the drug of choice in the treatment of serious infections with *Pseudomonas* species. Used in combination with amoxycillin and metronidazole, it forms the most commonly used combined treatment for life-threatening infections when the causative microbe is unknown. Other indications include the treatment of serious infections where laboratory tests show it to be the most effective agent. There will be very few indications for the use of gentamicin without the previous taking of a blood culture.

Dosage

Long experience has shown that the nomogram of Mawer enables one to compute accurately both loading and maintenance doses based on age, body weight in kg and blood creatinine. Blood creatinine needs to be repeated during therapy and the dose correspondingly modified (Ledward and Hawkins, 1983).

Control

In straightforward cases in young and middle-aged people with normal renal function, it is not necessary to control blood levels by laboratory tests. Such tests should, however, always be used in patients with abnormal renal function and in the aged whose excretion patterns may be irregular. Only rarely will a course of gentamicin need to be continued beyond five days.

Blood levels

At present blood levels are determined by a biological method using a range of microbes resistant to most antibacterial drugs apart from gentamicin. Some of the later cephalosporins cause us some difficulty so always, in every case, tell the laboratory precisely which antibiotics the patient is receiving. Tests are put up at noon and read late afternoon on the same day. Results can be telephoned. The recommended routine is, therefore:

a. Tell the laboratory the day before a test will be sent.
b. Take pre-dose blood 5 min before the dose.
c. Take post-dose blood:
    15 min after i.v. dosage.
    45 min after i.m. dosage.
d. Ensure that the blood reaches the laboratory before noon. If blood is not taken on the morning of the test, specimens can be satisfactorily stored overnight in the refrigerator.

Assay of Gentamicin

Blood levels are mandatory during treatment. Dosage of injections should be:

08:00–09:00 with the result ready before 17:00 to allow for the next dose to be determined.

The laboratory staff should be informed prior to requesting gentamicin assays.

CONGENITAL INFECTIONS

Sera from both *mother* and *baby* are important:

Syphilis
Toxoplasmosis
Rubella } Test are serological except herpes
Cytomegalovirus simplex
Herpes simplex

Remember these are often infectious to others.

ORGANISMS TRANSMITTED FROM MOTHER TO BABY

Some organisms that the mother can transmit to the baby at birth (and sometimes to the whole unit) are:

Haemolytic streptococci (particularly Group B)
Gonococci
Herpes simplex
Chlamydia
Chicken pox
Gastrointestinal infections.

Isolate first, ask questions afterwards, take samples.

FURTHER READING

Hawkins D. F. (1983) Drugs and pregnancy. In *Antimicrobial Drugs in Pregnancy*, Chap. 9, Ed. R. S. Ledward. Edinburgh, Churchill Livingstone

Ledward R. S. and Hawkins D. F. (1983) *Drug Treatment in Obstetrics.* London, Chapman & Hall.

Zuspan F. P. and Christian C. D. (1983) In *Controversy in Obstetrics and Gynaecology III*, Eds D. E. Reid and T. C. Barton, Chap. 16, pp. 450–476. London, W. B. Saunders

Chapter 19

Radiotherapy and Oncology

INTRODUCTION

These departments tend to be in specialized regional centres; junior medical staff should contact appropriate consultant colleagues to gain training.

TUMOUR MARKERS

Many forms of gynaecological cancer can now benefit by specialized treatment in addition to their primary surgery. Although chemotherapy often forms part of this treatment it is important not to use chemotherapy without careful consideration. Suboptimal use can prejudice the final outcome of treatment. This is particularly true of gestational choriocarcinoma and germ-cell tumours of the ovary. Specialized advice should always be sought since these tumours are potentially curable, however far advanced at diagnosis. Similar considerations now apply to many cases of ovarian epithelial cancer and advanced carcinoma of the cervix. Tumour markers are increasingly important in the management of gynaecological cancer:

Choriocarcinoma	HCG
Germ-cell tumours	HCG, AFP
Ovarian epithelial cancer	Carcinoembryonic antigen (CEA)

Tumour marker assays are available through the supra-regional assay services.

CYTOTOXIC THERAPY IN GYNAECOLOGY

See Ledward, 1984.

Carcinoma of Uterine Corpus

The use of progestogen therapy in the management of patients with carcinoma of the corpus is now established.

Carcinoma of the Ovary

Adriamycin cyclophosphamide; *cis*-platinum, chlorambucil and many other drugs have been used in the management of carcinoma in the ovary. No established dosage regime is available and many local variations of therapy will exist.

Chorionic Carcinoma

The place of methotrexate for chorionic carcinoma is established.

Cervical Carcinoma

No established cytotoxic drug is available. Adriamycin and methotrexate have been tried.

The haematological response to cytotoxic therapy should be charted.

PROTOCOL FOR TREATMENT OF OVARIAN CARCINOMA WITH ADRIAMYCIN AND CYCLOPHOSPHAMIDE (I.V.)

After extensive surgical excision of tumour, combined chemotherapy has been shown to have synergistic therapeutic effect on ovarian carcinoma.

Combination Cytotoxic Therapy
See Table 19.1.

Table 19.1. Combined chemotherapy, adriamycin and cyclophosphamide for ovarian carcinoma

Maximum 10 cycles, at 4-weekly intervals

Maximum adriamycin cumulative dose: 450 mg/m^2

Dosage: Adriamycin 30–40 mg/m^2
Cyclophosphamide 500 mg/m^2

Patient's name:

Diagnosis and staging:

Recommended dosage:

Initial investigation results: Full blood count: Liver function tests: ECG:

Comment

Cycle	1	2	3	4	5	6	7	8	9	10
Date:										
WBC:										
Platelets:										
Dose given:										
Cumulative adriamycin dose										
ECG (3 monthly)										
Buccal sensation										
Other side-effects, comments										

Dosage

Adriamycin   30–40 mg/m^2 ⎫ Single dose
Cyclophosphamide   500 mg/m^2 ⎬ treatment every
                                        ⎭ 3 or 4 weeks

a. Reduced dosage for:
  i.   Elderly   50% of
  ii. Previous chemotherapy   recommended
  iii. Impaired liver function   dosage

  Liver function tests

Serum bilirubin (mg/100 ml)	Adriamycin dosage (%)
1·2 (normal)	100
< 1·2–3·0	50
> 3·0	25

  iv. Myelosuppression

Blood count	Adriamycin dosage + cyclophosphamide (%)
White blood cells < 4000 Platelets ⩾ 130 000	100
White blood cells 3900–2900 Platelets 129 000–75 000	50
White blood cells < 2500 Platelets < 75 000	Wait for recovery Full blood count weekly

b. Maximum of *ten cycles* or cumulative adriamycin dose of 450–480 mg/m^2.
c. In remission or after maximum dose, intermittent mephalan + hexamthylmelamine + cyclophosphamide.

Administration

a. Chemotherapy given through rubber tubing of free-running intravenous injection, to reduce risk of thrombosis.

b. Injected over period of 2–3 min.
c. Intravenous anti-emetics 30 min before injection then 4-hourly when necessary.

Investigation regime
a. Before chemotherapy—ECG, full blood count, liver function tests.
b. Monthly, before cycle—full blood count, screen for buccal ulceration.
c. Three monthly—ECG.

Monitoring of Side-Effects
a. Cardiac effects
 Tachycardia and ECG changes.
 Therefore routine ECG before starting treatment and 3-monthly.
b. Marrow suppression
 Effects 10 days after administration.
 Therefore routine FBC
  RBC
  WBC } Repeat before each treatment cycle
  Platelets
c. Alopecia: can be reduced by cooling of scalp.
d. Buccal ulceration:
 Preceded by buccal burning sensation.
 Therefore routine questioning for buccal sensation.
e. Gastrointestinal effects
 Nausea, diarrhoea, vomiting $\rightarrow$ *i.v. anti-emetics before therapy*.
 Appetite suppression $\rightarrow$ usually resolves 3 days after administration.
f. Urine discoloration and cystitis
 Red urine after administration of adriamycin is harmless.
 Cyclophosphamide can induce cystitis.

HYDATIDIFORM MOLE

Where hydatidiform mole is diagnosed *pre-evacuation* (i.e. by ultrasound), blood should be taken and 3–5 ml of serum sent to the supraregional assay service for HCG measurement.

Fresh mole tissue (not fixed) is a valuable research material and, provided the histopathology department has all the tissue it requires for histopathology, Charing Cross Hospital, London might like to be informed and, if suitable, collection could be arranged. The mole should be kept *sterile* and can be stored temporarily in tissue culture medium (TC199), or kept dry, in a refrigerator (4°C).

Registration

Any patient with macroscopic evidence of histopathological diagnosis of hydatidatidiform mole (complete or partial mole, mole with fetus) should be *registered* under the DHSS/RCOG scheme as soon as possible after evacuation. Registration forms are available from the supraregional assay service. This complements, but does not replace, local hospital follow-up. Evacuation is generally best effected spontaneously or by suction or curettage. The use of pitocin should be kept to a minimum. A curettage may be necessary following primary evacuation, particularly if there is continued blood loss. In the event of recurrent or persistent per vaginum blood loss or other symptoms or doubts about management the appropriate reference centre will help (Appendix II).

It is important for the laboratory to receive a serum specimen within three weeks of evacuation of hydatidiform mole. Patients with persisting high values > 20000 IU/l of HCG more than three weeks after evacuation of mole may require urgent treatment to prevent uterine perforation. HCG results are sent to the consultant.

There is a 10% chance that a patient with hydatidiform mole will require chemotherapy for invasive mole or choriocarcinoma and these cases are almost all identified within 6 months of evacuation. Identification of those requiring chemotherapy is largely dependent on regular HCG assays which reflect trophoblastic activity and the registration scheme ensures regular HCG follow-up.

The patient should be advised as follows:

a. Hydatidiform mole is an abnormal pregnancy with a risk of requiring special treatment (chemotherapy) for invasive mole or choriocarcinoma subsequently in 10% of cases.

b. Once registered, the patient will receive instructions about urine and serum samples, together with a postal box and instructions from the reference centre.

c. Pregnancy must be avoided until the 'all-clear' is given (*see below*).

Follow-up is continued on patients for two years following evacuation of a classical hydatidiform mole. Urine samples for HCG estimations are normally requested by the laboratory every two weeks until normal HCG values are obtained. A serum sample is then requested to confirm normal values. Further serum samples are requested if HCG is still detected in serum. After normal serum values have been confirmed, urines only are requested every month till the end of one year post-evacuation, and then three monthly during the second year.

Where a patient is anxious to go ahead with a further pregnancy it is probably safe to allow this to proceed after HCG has been normal for *six months* on urine and has been confirmed on serum assay (the risk of choriocarcinoma occurring in the second year of follow-up after HCG has been normal for six months is less than 1:500).

After partial mole or hydatidiform degeneration, i.e. mole with recognizable fetal tissues, a six months' follow-up period is usually adequate unless early results indicate persisting activity, in which case a full two-year follow-up is recommended. Again, where a patient is anxious to go ahead with a further pregnancy this is reasonable after HCG values have been normal for six months.

Further estimations of HCG three weeks and three months after any pregnancy following classical hydatidiform mole are recommended because of a small increase in risk of choriocarcinoma in such patients at that time. In some cases the choriocarcinoma arises from the new pregnancy.

Oestrogen or progestogen preparations for contraceptive or other purposes taken between the evacuation of the mole and the return to normality of gonadotrophin values appears to *more than double the risk* of invasive mole or choriocarcinoma requiring drug therapy. It is suggested that these be avoided until HCG has become undetectable in serum, i.e. < 2 IU/l.

FURTHER READING

Drug and Therapeutics Bulletin (1983) Unwanted effects of anti-cancer drugs. Vol. 21, No. 12. London, Consumer Association

Ledward R. S. (1984) *Drug Treatment in Gynaecology.* London, Butterworths

Chapter 20

Radiography and Ultrasonography

DEPARTMENT OF RADIOLOGY

Most X-ray departments are fully staffed from 09:00–17:00 hours on weekdays; out of these hours, an emergency service is provided. Mobile facilities are available.

Ten-day Rule

Details of menstrual cycle, last menstrual period (LMP) and 'sterilization' operations (if any) for females should be entered. Irradiation of the female of child-bearing age has now acquired a medicolegal significance. X-ray examination for such females is only safely performed during menstruation or the first ten days of the menstrual cycle (in the absence of a sterilization procedure). X-rays performed after the first ten days of the menstrual cycle can only be undertaken when the clinician writes 'ignore' above the LMP. This rule applies even to patients taking oral contraceptives. The clinician thus acquires a medicolegal responsibility should pregnancy subsequently be shown to be present at the time of the X-rays.

It would be a kindness to inform female patients of child-bearing age that their X-ray examination will be performed within the first ten days of the menstrual cycle and to point out that the X-ray department will have to enquire into the dates of the LMP.

Examination Requests

Request cards and films are filed alphabetically and it is, therefore, important that the patient's name be legible and correctly spelt. The date of birth and the date, findings and place of previous X-ray examinations should be given.

State the part of the body you wish examined (e.g. chest, abdomen etc.) or procedure (e.g. barium meal, cholecystogram etc.). In general, intravenous contrast examinations should be performed before barium examinations on in-patients and, if both are required, a barium enema should precede a barium meal. Abdominal X-rays in pregnancy should be countersigned by the consultant.

Clinical Information

The relevant clinical findings (history and examination) are essential for meaningful interpretation of the films. The pertinent clinical findings should be briefly stated. A tentative clinical diagnosis should also be given, but it is more helpful to indicate what particular problem needs resolution. It is usually considered good practice to order an X-ray only when it will alter clinical management.

Follow-Up

On repeat X-ray cards please indicate if any further developments or firm diagnoses have been reached. A 'post-op. chest' request is a good opportunity to state briefly the operative findings as well as operative procedure and date of operation . . . and whether or not they confirmed pre-operative diagnosis!

Ward Radiography

The planning of investigations can save time, trouble and expense. Whenever possible X-rays should be performed in the department. Ward-portable films are often unsatisfactory, costly and time-consuming and should only be requested when the patient is not fit enough to attend the department. It is possible to obtain portable films of the chest and abdomen, but other parts of the body, such as the skull or spine are not suitable for ward radiography. Portable (ward) X-rays should be kept to a minimum.

Consent
Written consent must be obtained from patients who require lymphangiograms, venograms.

Preparation for X-ray
In-patients attending the department should have all clothing removed and be dressed in white gowns. Instructions for preparation of patients for particular X-ray examinations should be strictly adhered to. The patient should be told the time, date and required preparation at the time the appointment is made. Patients attending for X-ray should have an empty bladder.

Filing of Reports
The end-product of the department is in the radiologist's report. Every effort should be made to ensure that these are filed correctly in the notes. Radiographs are the property of the X-ray department and should be returned to file when not required.

Special X-ray Examinations
Chest X-rays
These are not performed routinely.

Abdominal Calculi

If the radiological confirmation of suspected stones is required, the definitive examination (cholecystogram or urography) should be requested rather than plain films. There is no point in arranging plain films prior to such an examination.

Intravenous Urogram

Restriction of fluids, except in cases of renal failure or myeloma, should be strictly adhered to. For morning appointments, no breakfast or drinks after midnight should be taken. Three Senokot tablets should be taken at bedtime the night before the examination. A blood urea level should be estimated prior to the procedure.

Hysterosalpingography

Hysterosalpingograms are usually performed without any preparation or anaesthetic. RMOs should receive instruction from the registrars before delegation of this procedure.

Lymphangiogram

Patent blue violet 2·5% mixed with an equal quantity of 1% lignocaine, 1 ml is injected subcutaneously into the medial 3 web spaces of each foot.

Barium Enema

A rectal examination and sigmoidoscopy should be undertaken initially.

Pelvimetry

The value of pelvimetry is questioned. Erect lateral radiographs can be requested for vaginal breech delivery or when cephalo-pelvic disproportion is considered.

ULTRASOUND DEPARTMENT

It must be stressed that full clinical information should be provided, including the LMP. It is essential that at the time of examination the patient has a full bladder. A radiographer measures the fetal biparietal diameter (BPD) for estimation of fetal age. The more general examinations of the uterus are undertaken by a radiologist. Ultrasound requests should be countersigned by a registrar.

Ultrasonography in Gynaecology

Ultrasonography is useful for confirmation of pregnancy, examination for retained products or ectopic pregnancy, localization of intra-uterine contraceptive device, examination of ovaries.

Ultrasonography in Obstetrics

During the last decade the use of diagnostic ultrasound in obstetrics has become a routine part of obstetric management. The applications of ultrasound in obstetrics are:

a. Fetal measurement.
b. Placentography.
c. Examination in early pregnncy.

It is essential to have full clinical information including the LMP. The patient should have a full bladder at the time of examination.

Fetal Measurements

Fetal measurements are undertaken (*a*) to establish fetal maturity (*b*) to monitor fetal growth.

A wide range of fetal measurements can be undertaken. In the early pregnancy crown–rump length measurements are taken. In the second and third trimester, biparietal diameters are measured. In addition, the head circumference, abdominal circumference and the lengths of the long bones can be measured.

Placentography

The main clinical indication for placentography is the investigation of antepartum haemorrhage. This could be done at any time during the pregnancy. Prior to the general availability of ultrasound, all the reliable techniques of placentography required exposure of the mother and fetus to ionizing radiation.

Ultrasound Examination in Early Pregnancy

It is possible by detailed ultrasound scanning to detect fetal abnormalities such as anencephaly, neural tube defects, obstructive nephropathy and exomphalos. Ultrasound examination is also useful in differentiating between a complete abortion and an incomplete abortion and will reduce the need for postabortion uterine curettage.

Fetal deaths can often be established by ultrasound examination.

FURTHER READING

Campbell S. (1969) The prediction of fetal maturity by ultrasonic measurement of the biparietal diameter. *J. Obstet. Gynaecol. Br. Commonw.* **76**, 603–609

Campbell S. (Ed.) (1983) Ultrasound in obstetrics and gynaecology, recent advances. In *Clinics in Obstetrics and Gynaecology*, Vol. 10. London, W. B. Saunders

Chapter 21

Gynaecological Surgery

INTRODUCTION

Cold Cases

Cold cases are admitted by the consultant concerned, direct to the gynaecology wards, two days pre-operatively for major cases, one day pre-operatively or on the day of surgery for minor cases.

Maximum outpatient assessments, e.g. chest X-rays, blood grouping, haemoglobin should be taken prior to admission.

Patients are admitted and clerked by the SHO, the necessary investigations instigated and the registrar informed. Consultants may be informed of any such admission by the registrar.

All laboratory results should be checked and signed by the RMO prior to filing; abnormal results should be brought to the attention of the registrar and consultant.

Emergency Cases

Emergency cases are admitted by the SHO and admitted to the beds of the consultant under whom they have previously been admitted or the consultant on duty for the day.

Patients who have previously been admitted should be admitted to the consultant 'on take' unless the new admission relates to a previous condition which had merited admission. The patient should then be admitted to the consultant under whom they had previously been admitted.

PRE-OPERATIVE PREPARATIONS

All Major Cases

General

Two Senokot tablets are given on the night of admission and a disposable enema prior to surgery.

Patients have a bath and abdominal and perineal shaving is undertaken.

HEPARIN PROPHYLAXIS The following patients should receive prophylactic heparin—given subcutaneously, heparin 5000 IU twice daily. Support stockings may also be used until actively mobile (Allan *et al.*, 1983; Turner *et al.*, 1984).

a. Patients with previous proven deep vein thrombosis or pulmonary embolism (a pre-operative chest radiograph and bilateral ascending phlebography should be considered).
b. Major surgery.
c. Obesity.
d. Malignancy.
e. Heavy smokers.
f. Patients over 40 years of age.
g. Patients with hyperlipidaemia.
h. If in doubt, e.g. chronic bronchitic patients.

ANTIBIOTIC PROPHYLAXIS Within the UK the use of metronidazole (2 g per rectum on the pre- and first post-operative day and 200 mg three times a day orally to follow) is advocated, whereas within the USA other broad-spectrum antibiotics, e.g. cephalosporins, in addition to metronidazole are used routinely.

The use of long-acting sulponamides, e.g. sulphameto-pyrazine, may be considered where indwelling catheter-ization will be required. Unfortunately, many urinary tract infections are not sensitive to sulphonamides and catheter specimens should still be sent for sensitivity testing. (Also *see* Chapter 18 and Keighley, 1983.)

PREPARATION IN THEATRE Patients may receive a brilliant green vaginal douche and are catheterized in theatre after the general anaesthetic pre-operatively.

Laparoscopy and Minor Cases

Two suppositories are given and the patient has a bath. Suprapubic shaving is undertaken for laparoscopies.

LAPAROSCOPY

The *indications* for laparoscopy are well documented. They include:

Diagnosis
Evaluation of symptoms
Surgical procedures may be performed via laparoscopy.

The *morbidity* of laparoscopy is likewise well documented and includes:

Complications of gas insufflation
Complications of trocar
Complications of tubal diathermy.

Laparoscopy should *only be performed:*

By a practitioner of minimum registrar grade.
SHOs may be taught the procedure but the registrar must accept full responsibility.
No sterilization should be undertaken by a practitioner of less than registrar grading.

Previous abdominal surgery may be a relative contraindication depending on the experience of the practitioner.

DAY CASE PROCEDURES

Such procedures may include termination of pregnancy, cauterizing the cervix, insertion of intra-uterine contraceptive devices, D & C. All appropriate investigations should be performed usually as an outpatient procedure prior to the operation. In particular, haemoglobin and blood groups for termination patients should be requested at the clinic consultation. (*See* Saunders and Rowland, 1972.)

Procedure

a. Patients should arrive one hour prior to surgery.

b. Patients should have fasted for 8 hours, preferably from the previous midnight.

c. A friend or relative *must* collect the patient when they are ready to travel. Patients having very minor procedures under local anaesthetic are the only exceptions.

d. Patients having a general anaesthetic should rest for at least 3·5 hours post-operatively unless written directions to the contrary are left by the consultant.

e. Following anaesthetic patients *should not* drive a car or operate any kind of machinery.

f. It is recommended that patients should:

    i.   *Not* be diabetics taking insulin.

    ii. *Not* have a significant degree of respiratory disease.

    iii. *Not* have a significant degree of cardiac disease.

    iv. *Not* be hypertensive.

    v.   *Not* be taking steroid or monoamine oxidase drugs.

OPERATION LISTS

Date   *Surgeon's name*

Anaesthetist's name   *Time*

Patient's surname, forename   *Hospital No.*   *Age*

Proposed Operation—avoiding abbreviations

Remarks column Hb and LMP if relevant

Sickling Neg. or Pos.

Medical Conditions, e.g. Diabetes, Myasthenia gravis, TB and Heart
    conditions

Drugs which the patient may be taking

Any skeletal conditions relative to positioning, e.g. fixed and pinned
    joints, disc lesions etc.

Operation lists should *be delivered to the theatre office*
on the evening prior to the proposed list; minimal modifications should be required.

If instruments, other than those carried in the department are likely to be required, e.g. resection or vascular
trays, maximum warning should be given.

Emergency Operations

Medical staff should inform theatre and bring a completed
collection slip to the theatre.

For emergency additions to lists, e.g. evacuation of
retained products of conception, the SHO already working
in theatre will usually carry out these procedures, but it is
basic good manners for the SHO adding 'the case' to ask
his/her colleague. This also applies to the anaesthetist.

'Dirty cases' should be put at the end of the list.

Blood, whether it is required or for 'standby', is the
responsibility of the medical staff.

PATHOLOGY REQUESTS FROM THEATRE

For *all* specimens of body tissue, body fluids, urine, blood and pus, *a Pathology Request card MUST be completed by a member of the medical staff. This also applies to cytology requests.* (*See* Chapter 15.)

The request card must contain: patient's name, age, hospital number, consultant's name, together with type of material and the area of body from which it was taken. Last menstrual period and relevant information must also be supplied.

If more than one specimen is taken, but only one request card used, specimens must be listed.

Specific tests required should be indicated.

Urgent Specimens

These will be taken directly to the laboratory, provided they are covered by a completed request form marked 'Urgent'.

No specimen will be accepted by the laboratory unless clearly labelled and the specimen and request card correspond.

Forms must be completed no later than the end of the list.

Special Requests

For example, frozen sections can usually be undertaken provided the *medical staff make the necessary arrangements with the laboratory and theatre.*

Sterilizations

Many methods are available (p. 106) but if a tubal ligation is performed then samples of fallopian tube should be sent for histological examination.

Curettings

Curettings should be sent in saline (for exclusion of tuberculosis) and in formalin (for histological examination) in cases of infertility.

POST-OPERATIVE MANAGEMENT

All patients should be seen on the first post-operative day to assess:

a. Fluid balance—a good urine output should be confirmed following hysterectomy.

b. Vital signs: temperature, pulse etc.

c. Analgesia—the initial post-operative analgesia will be prescribed by the anaesthetist, further analgesia will be supervised by the SHO (Twycross, 1977).

d. Psychotherapy—a full explanation of the surgical procedure should be given to the patient as soon as convenient.

e. Assess potential complications:

    i. Haemorrhage—2 units of blood should be available prior to surgery where blood loss can be anticipated.

    ii. Infection—a post-operative pyrexia within 24 hours does not necessarily call for antibiotics.

    iii. Deep vein thrombosis treatment—anticoagulant control (*see below*).

    iv. Post-operative embolism—appropriate management is indicated in *Fig.* 21.1.

Anticoagulant Control

Anticoagulant therapy in gynaecological patients should be along the lines indicated by *Fig.* 21.1 and the information provided below. The following regime is recommended for starting patients on anticoagulants: warfarin sodium is the

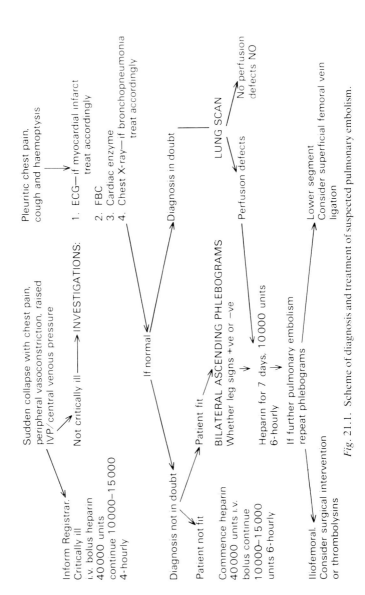

Fig. 21.1. Scheme of diagnosis and treatment of suspected pulmonary embolism.

drug of first choice (with or without immediate heparinization). A single large dose is given initially, the size of which varies with age, body weight, degree of illness. In general, old or very ill or very small people require smaller initial doses; younger, heavier or relatively fit people should have higher initial doses. The recommended doses shown in *Table* 16.1 (p. 157) are average and should be adjusted in accordance with considerations.

When a patient is to be discharged on anticoagulant treatment, notify the haematology laboratory in good time by sending the anticoagulant card with the section headed 'Request for Outpatient Control' completed.

OUTPATIENT FOLLOW-UP APPOINTMENTS

Excessive follow-up appointments should be restricted; a guide may be provided by referral to *Table* 12.1, p. 125.

FURTHER READING

Allan A., Williams J. T., Bolton J. P. *et al.* (1983) The use of graduated compression stockings in the prevention of post-operative deep vein thrombosis. *Br. J. Surg.* **70**, 172–174

Keighley M. R. B. (1983) Perioperative antibiotics. *Br. Med. J.* **286**, 1844–1845

Saunders P. and Rowland R. (1972) Vacuum curettage of the uterus without anaesthesia. *J. Obstet. Gynaecol. Br. Commonw.* **79**, 168–174

Turner G. M. and Brooks J. H. (1984) The efficacy of graduated compression stockings in the prevention of deep vein thrombosis after major gynaecological surgery. *Br. J. Obstet. Gynaecol.* **91**, 588–591

Twycross R. G. (1977) Choice of analgesics in terminal cancer. *Practitioner,* **219**, 475–478

Chapter 22

Pharmaceutical Services

INTRODUCTION

The house officer will initially be acquiring his new skills as an accomplished accoucheur and gynaecological resident. In obstetric practice, minimum prescribing of drugs should be the norm and to assist the SHO the services of the clinical pharmacist on the weekly 'Grand Rounds' is most advantageous; advice as to particular drug preparations, costs, incompatibilities is then immediately at hand and the house officer can then supervise the drug charts with added vigilance.

CLINICAL SERVICES

Pharmacists visit each ward daily to review treatment charts. Pharmacists also join some consultant ward rounds. The SHO should use these visits as an opportunity to discuss any queries or problems related to drug therapy (*see* Leach *et al.*, 1981; Cairns and Prior, 1983; Jones *et al.*, 1984; Gibson and Freebron, 1985).

Particular areas in which pharmacists may be able to offer useful advice are: choice of medications, based on the patient's clinical condition; adverse effects; drug interactions and their clinical implications; interpretation of drug plasma levels; methods of formulating drugs and availability and supply of drug products.

198

DRUG INFORMATION

A drug information centre is usually based within the pharmacy department.

THERAPEUTIC DRUG MONITORING

The pharmacy department, in collaboration with the clinical chemistry department, may offer a therapeutic drug monitoring service for the following drugs: digoxin, gentamicin, theophylline, phenytoin, phenobarbitone, primidone, carbamazepine and lithium. Details of such a service and advice on optimal sampling times may be obtained from either department.

It is important to add full clinical details, the dosage regimen, the time of last dose and sampling time to the request form, as all this information is vital to the interpretation of the level.

NOTES ON THE USE OF DRUG PRESCRIPTIONS

a. The patient's name, ward and registration details must be on the card.
b. A prescription sheet will have several sections:
     i. Regularly administered prescriptions.
     ii. Once only and pre-medication drugs.
     iii. Variable dose and as required prescriptions.
     iv. Drugs to take away.

Prescriptions should be entered in the *appropriate* section of the chart.

All prescriptions should be written clearly in *block capitals*.

c. The following information is required:
  i. Approved name: the proprietary name should only be used if the preparation is a mixture of several drugs.
  ii. Dose of drug: the dose should be expressed precisely. Abbreviations such as mg, ml, may be used, but for doses expressed in micrograms, the word micrograms should be written in full, to avoid any confusion between the abbreviations mg and mcg.
  iii. Route of administration: this must be clearly stated. If an eyedrop is prescribed, please indicate which eye is to receive medication. For dermatological preparations, please indicate the area of the body to which the preparation is to be applied.
  iv. Time of administration: for regular prescriptions, if the time is not indicated, the 'recommended times for administration' in the central section of the prescription sheet will be adopted by the nursing staff.

   Antibiotics should always be prescribed in terms of dosage interval rather than number of doses to be given per day. This ensures an optimal dosage regime is adopted and subtherapeutic serum levels avoided.
  v. The date on which treatment is to be initiated.
  vi. The prescriber's signature.

d. Cancellation or alterations to prescriptions—when a prescription is cancelled, a line should be drawn through it and the 'cancellation' section signed and dated by the prescriber. If the dosage or route of administration is *altered*, the original prescription should be *cancelled* and *rewritten*.

e. If the patient is known to be sensitive or allergic to any drug, this information should be entered on the front of the sheet in the appropriate section.

f. Parenteral fluid therapy—the prescriber must enter details of every bottle, plus additives if appropriate, on the chart. The date and time of termination of treatment must be clearly indicated. It is not sufficient to write the frequency of administration only.

g. Anticoagulant therapy—a separate chart is available for recording anticoagulant therapy. Reference should be made to this chart on the prescription sheet. For example, 'Warfarin—*see* separate sheet'. The two sheets should be kept together on the ward.

h. Prescriptions for drugs to take home—write up prescriptions to take home well in advance of the date of discharge, in order to prevent unnecessary delay and inconvenience to patients when leaving hospital. Normally, not more than fourteen days' treatment should be prescribed.

i. Prescribing of controlled drugs and barbiturates—the prescription must comply fully with the requirements of the Misuse of Drugs Act 1973. The following requirements apply to prescriptions for out-patients and drugs to take home. For in-patients there are no special requirements for prescriptions for controlled drugs:

    i. The entire prescription must be in the prescriber's own handwriting in ink or another indelible agent.

    ii. The prescription must bear:

        The name and address of the patient.

        The date.

        The prescriber's full signature (not initials).

        The form of the preparations (e.g. tablets, linctus etc.), and the strength (e.g. 5 mg tablets).

        The dose to be taken.

        Either the total quantity of the preparation, or the total number of dosage units to be supplied. This must be written in words and figures.

INTRAVENOUS ADDITIVES

Wherever possible, the addition of drugs to intravenous fluids should be carried out under aseptic conditions in the pharmacy department. If an intravenous additive is required out of pharmacy hours, the physician should contact a pharmacist through the switchboard.

If an additive is needed urgently and must be prepared on the ward, the following points should be noted:

a. Drugs should not generally be added to the following solutions: blood or blood products; fat emulsions; dextrans; mannitol; sodium bicarbonate; amino acid solutions; Hartmann's solution.

b. No more than one drug should be added to an infusion fluid.

c. Valuable advice on the preparation of intravenous additives can be found in the British National Formulary. Further advice on incompatibilities or stability of prepared infusions may be obtained by contacting a pharmacist.

Special Situations

Antibiotics

The addition of antibiotics to large volumes of intravenous fluids may result in subtherapeutic serum levels; thus most antibiotics should be given by intravenous bolus. Exceptions to this rule are: erythromycin, fusidic acid, amphotericin, miconazole. For these drugs, intravenous bolus injection may result in phlebitis or vein collapse.

Potassium

Potassium is commercially available in concentrations of 20 and 40 mmol/l, in the following infusion fluids: dextrose 5%; dextrose 4% + saline 0·18%; saline 0·9%. If other concentrations of potassium are required, they should be requested from the pharmacy.

HAEMATINICS

The following are in common use: ferrous salts, total dose iron dextran (Imferon) infusion, strong compound vitamin B, folic acid.

Oral Iron Therapy in Pregnancy

In iron deficiency states a total daily dose of 100–200 mg of elemental iron should be prescribed (Ledward and Hawkins, 1983). The following iron salts are to be prescribed wherever possible:

Iron preparation		Elemental iron/tablet
Ferrous sulphate	200 mg	60 mg
Ferrous gluconate	300 mg	35 mg
Ferrous fumarate	200 mg	65 mg

If the patient experiences side-effects, the dose should be reduced or an alternative iron salt prescribed.

Slow release iron preparations e.g. Feospan, are designed to release elemental iron gradually as the dosage form passes through the gut; however, as iron is only absorbed to any degree in the first part of the duodenum, the reduced incidence of side-effects associated with slow release preparations usually reflects reduced iron absorption. Slow release iron preparations thus offer no therapeutic advantage and are also considerably more expensive than simple ferrous salts.

The addition of ascorbic acid to iron preparations in order to increase iron absorption has been shown to be of minimal therapeutic advantage in the concentrations available commercially and products containing such combinations (e.g. Ferrograd C) have now been 'black-listed' and cannot be prescribed under the NHS.

Many other combinations of iron with multivitamins, minerals or folic acid have also been blacklisted. Check with pharmacy or a copy of the 'blacklist' if there is doubt as to whether a preparation can be prescribed.

The Total Dose Iron-Dextran Technique (TDI)

Procedure

a. Determine the patient's requirements of iron dextran (Imferon) from the dosage table. This shows the total volume of iron dextran necessary to restore the haemo-globin level to normal and replenish the reserve and tissue iron. In pregnancy an additional 10 ml (= 500 mg Fe) should be added to meet the demands of the fetus and to compensate for blood loss at delivery.

b. The infusion should be prepared in the pharmacy. The resultant iron dextran solution will not exceed 5% iron dextran vol./vol.

c. Ensure that facilities are available for the emergency treatment of shock (*see below*).

d. Before venepuncture the skin should be cleansed with methylated spirit only. A test-dose should be given at a rate not exceeding 5 drops/min for 10 minutes under strict medical supervision. If this test-dose is well tolerated the rate of infusion may be increased to 45–60 drops/min.

e. Outpatients should be kept under supervision for about an hour after the infusion is complete before returning home.

Response

Following TDI there is usually a rapid rise in the haemo-globin level. This is most marked during the first two weeks after treatment and is directly related to the severity of the anaemia. Thereafter, there is a further gradual rise until the haemoglobin reaches normality.

During the first 4 weeks, an average of 1 g haemoglobin per 100 ml (7%) per week can be expected.

Reaction

Anaphylactoid reactions can occur almost immediately after commencement of the infusion. *The drip should be changed to normal saline with a new set and treatment of shock instituted as follows:*

a. Chlorpheniramine i.v.
b. Hydrocortisone 100 mg stat i.v.
c. Oxygen.
d. Adrenaline (1 ml × 1/10000) should be drawn up ready prior to commencing infusion.

Post-infusion allergic type reactions have been reported. These respond quickly to appropriate therapy. Transient local phlebitis may occur at the site of the venepuncture which may require anti-inflammatory measures.

OTHER PHARMACEUTICAL SERVICES

Although not often required on obstetrics and gynaecological wards, pharmacy does also provide a total parenteral nutrition service and a cytotoxic reconstitution service.

FURTHER READING

Cairns C. J. and Prior F. G. R. (1983) The clinical pharmacist: a study of his hospital involvement. *Pharmaceut. J.* **229**, 16–18

Gibson P. and Freebron S. F. (1985) Are pharmacists effective on clinical rounds? *Pharmaceut. J.* **231**, 201–202

Jones A. N., Benzie R. L., Serjeant C. S. and Swan G. T. (1984) Activities of clinical pharmacists at ward level. *Aust. J. Hosp. Pharm.* **14**, 77–81

Leach R. H., Feetam C. and Butler D. (1981) An evaluation of a ward pharmacy service. *J. Clin. Hosp. Pharm.* **6**, 173–182

Ledward R. S. (1984) *Drug Treatment in Gynaecology.* London, Butterworths

Ledward R. S. and Hawkins D. F. (1983) *Drug Treatment in Obstetrics.* London, Chapman & Hall

Chapter 23

Clinical Budgeting

INTRODUCTION

Good health is an expensive product and the economics of good health could be introduced into undergraduate and postgraduate programmes. In recent years the concept of clinical budgeting has been introduced into practice.

THE GRIFFITHS REPORT—GENERAL MANAGEMENT

Clinical budgeting is a concept which was given widespread national significance by the publication of the Griffiths Management Inquiry Report in Autumn 1983. Griffiths was invited by DHSS Ministers to head a small review group charged with examining management processes in the health service. They recommended the introduction of general managers at health authority and hospital level to lead what had hitherto been consensus management teams. Furthermore they felt that doctors, who are the primary initiators of expenditure in the health service, should be given more responsibility for the resources they commit—that they should hold clinical budgets.

EARLIER DEVELOPMENTS IN CLINICAL BUDGETING

The idea of clinical budgeting was not entirely new to the NHS in 1983, since a number of experiments were already underway seeking to involve doctors more closely in planning and budgeting for the services they provide.

FINANCIAL SYSTEMS

The development of clinical budgeting has been hindered to some extent by the traditional health service financial systems. These are organized on a 'functional' basis, i.e. we know how much is spent each year on nursing, pharmacy, radiology, medical staffing, but we do not know how much we spend on a surgical programme or an obstetrics programme.

Before we can begin to ask surgeons or obstetricians to take on responsibility for a budget for the service they provide, we must develop systems which enable us to know what quantity of resources they are actually using. The rapid development of computer technology has made a significant contribution to our ability to produce accurate and timely expenditure reports. We can now identify how much it costs to treat a given number of surgical or obstetric patients over a given period of time. We can then estimate future need and future costs in consultation with clinicians and agree a prospective clinical budget.

THE ATTITUDE OF THE MEDICAL PROFESSION

In common with most Western countries, in recent years the British health service has seen a deceleration in the pace of growth after the relative 'boom' years of the 1960s and early 1970s. With growing awareness of resource constraints (particularly in the acute hospital sector as successive governments have been committed to the growth of traditionally underprivileged services for the elderly, mentally ill and mentally handicapped), the medical profession has become more convinced of the need to participate in some of the difficult decisions on how limited resources should best be spent. There has, recently, been guarded support for the development of clinical budgeting from most of the main professional organizations—guarded, because the associations are also aware of the need to preserve the doctor's responsibility to give the best care possible to his individual patients. Inevitably, on occasion there will be inherent conflict between management responsibility assumed through the acceptance of a clinical budget and clinical responsibility to a particular patient or group of patients. It is in the resolution of such conflicts that the future of clinical budgeting will, successful or otherwise, be determined.

SUMMARY

The house officer or registrar may not initially consider clinical budgeting his priority duty; it is, however, a part responsibility that he must bear as a member of the team and the SHO should be alert to the potential expense of unnecessary prescribing or investigations. It could be best considered that the SHO should give his patient his best possible care—leaving the discussion relating to unnecessary prescribing or investigations to the teaching ward round with the registrar and/or consultant.

FURTHER READING
Health Service Management (1984) *Implementation of the NHS Management Inquiry Report.* HC (84) 13. London, DHSS

Appendices

Weight Conversion Chart

kg	stone lbs		kg	stone lbs		kg	stone lbs		kg	stone lbs	
50	7	12	62·5	9	11·5	72·5	11	5·5	82·5	12	13·5
51	8	0·25	63	9	12·5	73	11	6·5	83	13	0·5
52	8	2·5	63·5	9	13·75	73·5	11	7·75	83·5	13	1·75
53	8	4·5	64	10	0·75	74	11	8·75	84	13	2·75
54	8	6·75	64·5	10	2	74·5	11	10	84·5	13	4
55	8	9	65	10	3	75	11	11	85	13	5
55·5	8	10	65·5	10	4	75·5	11	12	86	13	7·25
56	8	11·5	66	10	5·25	76	11	13·25	87	13	9·5
56·5	8	12·25	66·5	10	6·25	76·5	12	0·25	88	13	11·5
57	8	13·5	67	10	7·5	77	12	1·5	89	13	13·75
57·5	9	0·5	67·5	10	8·5	77·5	12	2·5	90	14	2
58	9	1·5	68	10	9·5	78	12	3·5	91	14	4·75
58·5	9	2·75	68·5	10	10·75	78·5	12	4·75	92	14	6·5
59	9	3·75	69	10	11·75	79	12	5·75	93	14	8·5
59·5	9	5	69·5	10	13	79·5	12	7	94	14	10·75
60	9	6	70	11	0	80	12	8	95	14	13
60·5	9	7	70·5	11	1	80·5	12	9	96	15	1·75
61	9	8·25	71	11	2·25	81	12	10·25	97	15	3·5
61.5	9	9·75	71·5	11	3·25	81·5	12	11·25	98	15	5·5
62	9	10·5	72	11	4·5	82	12	12·5	90	15	7·75

Supraregional Assay Service

All the following assays are available through the Supraregional Assay Service. Samples should be sent to the laboratories listed in the *Assay Service Handbook* which has been sent to all hospital chemical pathology departments by arrangements with the local chemical pathologist. He/she will also advise on the nature of the sample required and the range of normal values. Where there is likely to be a regular demand for a particular assay, it is suggested that the clinician or chemical pathologist concerned should enquire whether special arrangements would be advantageous.

ACTH	Belfast
	Newcastle
	St Bartholomew's
	St Thomas's
α-Fetoprotein (AFP)	Belfast
	Charing Cross
Calcitonin	Hammersmith
Carcinoembryonic antigen (CEA)	Charing Cross
	Glasgow
Ferritin	Cardiff

HGB and HCGB	Charing Cross
	Sheffield (Jessop Hospital)
	Dundee
Ovarian antigen CX_1	Charing Cross
Placental alkaline phosphatase	Charing Cross

Postgraduate Training and Examinations

Junior staff are encouraged to read and enter examinations for the higher diplomas:

1. DRCOG   Regulations from:
   Royal College of Obstetricians and
   Gynaecologists
   27 Sussex Place, Regent's Park,
   London NW1 4RG.

2. FRCS(Ed.) Regulations from:
   Royal College of Surgeons
   Nicholson Street, Edinburgh 8.

3. MRCP(Lond.) Regulations from:
   Royal College of Physicians
   11 St Andrew's Place,
   London NW1 4LE.

4. Postgraduate courses are held at the Royal College of Obstetricians and Gynaecologists, and the Institute of Obstetrics and Gynaecology at Queen Charlotte's Maternity Hospital, Goldhawk Road, London W6.

5. Diploma in Human Sexuality:
   St George's Hospital Medical School
   Postgraduate Office
   Cranmer Terrace, London SW17 0RE (01-672-1255 Ext 4499).

6. Diploma in Psychosexual Medicine:
   Margaret Pyke Centre
   15 Bateman Building
   Soho Square
   London W1V 5PW (01-734-9351).

Local courses normally available in Obstetrics and Gynaecology include:

   Perinatal meetings
   Journal clubs
   DRCOG lectures
   MRCOG lectures
   Postgraduate lectures
   and
   postgraduate tutorials

Junior staff are encouraged to keep details of cases suitable for the MRCOG examination: to publish papers of clinical importance and undertake minor research programmes after consultation with their consultants. A full record of their work is required for college recognition prior to taking the MRCOG examination.

The following societies should also be contacted for details of postgraduate training:

The British Society of Colposcopy and Cervical Pathology
Department of Obstetrics and Gynaecology,
Ninewells Hospital,
Dundee DD1 9SY
(0382-60111 Ext 2147)

The British Obstetric Computer Society
Department of Obstetrics and Gynaecology,
University Hospital,
Queens Medical Centre,
Nottingham NG7 2UH
(0602-700111 Ext 4180)

The Obstetrical Anaesthesia Society
Department of Anaesthetics,
Bristol Maternity Hospital,
Southwell Street,
Bristol BS2 8EG
(0272-22041)

The Blair Bell Research Society
Academic Department of Obstetrics and Gynaecology,
Royal Free Hospital,
Pond Street,
London NW3 2QG
(01-749-0500 Ext 3736)

The Royal Society of Medicine
1 Wimpole Street,
London W1M 8AE
(01-580-2070)

The Royal College of Obstetricians and Gynaecologists
27 Sussex Place,
Regent's Park,
London NW1 4RG
(01-262-5425)

The British Medical Ultrasound Society
36 Portland Place,
London W1N 3DG
(01-636-3714)

The British Medical Laser Association
Ear, Nose and Throat Department,
Royal South Hants Hospital,
Graham Road,
Southampton SO9 4EP
(0703-34288 Ext 214)

The Medical Society for the Study of Venereal Diseases
Department of Genito-Urinary Medicine,
General Infirmary,
Great George Street,
Leeds,
W. Yorkshire LS1 3EX
(0532-432799 Ext 2112)

The British Association of Social Psychiatry
112a Harley Street,
London W1N 1AF
(01-935-7776)

The Family Planning Association
27–35 Mortimer Street,
London W1N 7RJ
(01-636-7866)

The Society for the Study of Fertility
141 Newmarket Road,
Cambridge CB5 8HA
(0223-351810)

The College of Health
18 Victoria Park Square,
London E2
(01-980-6263)

Emergency Obstetric Service

'Flying Squad' Equipment

Pack

Delivery and suture pack
Hibitane cream
Savlon
Gloves
Amnihook
Plastic apron
Incontinence pads } Packed in box
Urinary catheter
Razor
Raytep gauze
Cottonwool balls
Crepe bandage
Pudendal block needle
Catgut

Box with

i.v. cannula
Syringes—varying sizes
Needles—varying sizes
Medicated swabs
Blood bottles—Hb + X-match
Elastic adhesive bandage
Micropore
Tourniquet
Small airstrips

Sphygmomanometer + stethoscope
Airway
Ambubag and facemask
Simms & Cusco speculum
Post AN set
Intravenous cutdown set—adult and child
Dripstand
Intravenous administration sets—blood and fluids
Three-way tap stopcock
Airway set for i.v. fluid

Intravenous Fluids
Dextrose/saline 1000 ml
5% dextrose 1000 ml
Hartmann's solution, 1000 ml
1 N saline 1000 ml
Haemacel, 500 ml
Sodium bicarbonate 8·4% 200 ml
Pinard's stethoscope

Bag with
Penlon
Facemask—sucker × 1—funnel × 1
Laryngoscope
Airway size 00
Extra batteries and bulb for laryngoscope
Mucous extractor
Syringes 10 + 2 + 1 ml
Orange needles
Mediswab
Surgical blade
Infants' resuscitation set size 10 and 12
Metal introducer
Portable manual suction machine
Yankours oral catheter

Drugs for Use

Adrenaline injection, 1 mg in 1 ml
Phenergan injection 25 mg in 1 ml
Hydrocortisone sodium succinate injection, 100 mg
Neonatal naloxone hydrochloride, 2-ml ampoules
Lignocaine 1% in 10 ml
* Amyl nitrate 0·3 ml in vitrellae
* Ergometrine injection 500 μg (mcg) in 1 ml
* Oxytocin, 2 units
* Oxytocin + ergometrine (Syntometrine)
  1-ml ampoules
Pethidine 100 mg 2 ampoules × 2
Diazepam, 10 mg 3 ampoules × 2

* These drugs are obtained from the refrigerator.

Notes for Guidance to those seeking Permission for Postmortem Examinations

The obtaining of consent for postmortem examination from bereaved relatives is clearly a delicate task, requiring great sensitivity, and is one in which the greatest care must be taken not to cause unnecessary distress.

It is necessary for those 'in lawful possession of the body'—normally the Area Health Authority or their designated agent (e.g. hospital secretary)—to obtain permission for a postmortem examination from the relatives of the deceased. In compliance with the Human Tissue Act, authorization may be given by those in lawful possession of the body for the medical staff to remove such tissues as may be deemed necessary for therapeutic purposes or for the purpose of medical education or research, provided that after reasonable enquiry there is no reason to believe that:

a. The deceased had expressed an objection to his body being so dealt with after death.
b. The surviving spouse or any surviving relative of the deceased objects to the body being so dealt with.

In practice, the medical staff use their professional discretion on the extent of each individual postmortem examination.

It may be helpful to summarize some of the important reasons for undertaking postmortem examinations.

Accuracy of Diagnosis

The pathologist is often able to establish with greater accuracy the precise diagnosis of the major illness, and also to correlate any complicating factors and other disease processes which may be present. Samples of tissue for further examination (e.g. microscopic, chemical, micro-biological etc.) may be taken.

Accuracy of Certification and Classification of Disease

Surveys of death certificates correlated with autopsy findings often reveal inaccuracies in certification. Much statistical information regarding the overall planning of health care resources, epidemiological information and other important factors, relies on the Registrar General's figures produced by death certification and it is imperative that these be as accurate as possible.

Educational Aspects

The bank of knowledge and experience obtained from postmortem examination is of considerable benefit to all patients in the future:

a. Via the pathologist: by increasing his understanding of the various disease processes that he will encounter in living patients he is able to give better advice to his clinical colleagues.

b. Via clinicians, radiologists etc.: the study of postmortem findings enables them to correlate their own investigations with the actual disease process. This adds considerably, and in a progressively cumulative manner, to their own expertise both in the fields of diagnosis and treatment.

c. Via undergraduate and postgraduate students: they will be learning about disease, either for the first time, or they are continuing their medical education throughout their career. It is essential that they have access to pathological material.

Therapeutic Aspects

The possibility of using certain tissues or organs for the treatment of living patients is a relatively recently introduced aspect.

a. *Organs for transplantation purposes are obtained by a special, separate procedure and do not form the subject matter for this Handbook.*

b. *Extracts from certain organs* can be prepared for the treatment of patients, e.g. pituitary extract. This helps two main groups of patients.

    i. *Children* who are suffering from a form of dwarfism. These patients are small in number, but if not treated they would not grow properly and would remain as dwarfs. They are usually detected at the age of 3 or 4 years and treatment (one injection two or three times per week of pituitary growth hormone) has to be continued throughout the entire growth phase until puberty. The hormone has to be of *human* type and no animal product or synthetic form can be used. The extraction process is difficult and expensive. It is carried out in this country by the Medical Research Council and the treatment of all patients is well controlled. The United Kingdom is unique in having a national programme for the collection of glands and for the provision of this drug and it would be a tragedy for this fine scheme to be jeopardized. The Medical Research Council controls the standard of material produced, and to some extent its use is still in an experimental stage. It is thus most important to have one group controlling the quality of the substance. The Medical

Research Council does not give money for the purchase of the glands, but a small honorarium is paid to the mortuary technician for the extra work involved in the preservation and dispatch of the gland.

ii. *Subfertile women* can be helped in some cases by treatment with follicle-stimulating hormone from the pituitary gland. The human gland is an important source, but unlike the growth hormone it is not the only source. The alternative source is the extraction of the hormone from urine.

The hormone is given over a period of about a week once a month, over a period of several months.

REQUESTS FOR POSTMORTEM EXAMINATIONS

From the above notes it will be clear that the request to relatives for a postmortem examination is made '*to learn more about the disease which caused the death of the deceased for the sake of others*' rather than to find out why the patient died. The new consent forms have been worded in order to convey this attitude, and to meet the requirements of the Human Tissue Act (p. 60).

REQUEST FOR POSTMORTEM EXAMINATION:

Hospital	*Ward*	*Surname*	*Reg. No.*
Doctor Requesting		*First Name*	*D.O.B.*
Date and Time of Death		*Address*	
Consultant		*G.P.*	

Has the Coroner Been Informed:
Is the Subject an Infective Risk:
(e.g. TB, AA+ etc. please give details)

Major Clinical Problems, Including Trauma, Operations and Treatment

(1)
(2)
(3)
(4)
(5)
(6)

Death Certificate Diagnosis: I *(a)*   II
                                      (b)
                                      (c)

Any Specific Information Sought:

History of Terminal Events:

Signed

Date

Stillbirths

The resident or midwife should write in the patient's notes:

1. Whether stillborn certificate has been signed and by whom.
2. If postmortem is required.
3. If doctor has arranged the postmortem.
4. Consent for postmortem signed.
5. If hospital or patient is burying the baby.
6. If hospital burial, details concerning disposal certificate.

Guidelines for the Training of Male Student Nurses

1. Clinical teaching must be arranged only with full consent of the patient, who should clearly understand that the observer is a student nurse.
2. As with female student nurses, observation of delivery should be part of the training, but only with the full consent of the patient and her husband. Aspects of abnormal delivery may be introduced under some safeguard.
3. Care should be taken at all times that the male student nurse is not permitted to be alone with the patient in circumstances which might lead to misinterpretation of the purpose of his presence.
4. Any nursing which might involve intimate care will depend on local circumstances and attitudes and the degree of cooperation of the individual patient.

Useful Telephone Numbers

Consultant Obstetricians

    1.
    2.
    3.
    4.
    5.
    6.
    7.
    8.

Consultant Paediatricians

    1.
    2.
Secretary 3.

Consultant Haematologist

    1.
MLSO   2.
Secretary 3.

Consultant Biochemist

        1.
MLSO   2.
Secretary 3.

Consultant Histopathologist

        1.
MLSO   2.
Secretary 3.

Consultant Microbiologist

        1.
MLSO   2.
Secretary 3.

Principal Pharmacist

        1.

Consultant Radiologists

        1.
        2.
        3.
Secretary

Consultant Radiotherapist

        1.
Secretary

Miscellaneous

1.
2.
3.
4.
5.
6.
7.
8.
9.
10.

INDEX

Abortion 129–39
  first trimester, curettage 132, 136
  incomplete, management 131, 132
    procedure 131, 132
  missed, prostaglandin use 135, 136
  recurrent
    investigations 133, 134
    primary and secondary 135
    treatment 134
  second trimester 136–8
  septic 138
  therapeutic
    forms 136
    patient preparation 137
    prostaglandin use 137, 138
  threatened, management 129, 130
Adrenal gland disorders, management 13, 14
Adriamycin
  ovarian cancer 175–9
  side-effects 179
Adverse reactions
  adriamycin 179
  cyclophosphamide 179
  iron 203
  prostaglandins 67
  salbutamol 60
  total dose iron–dextran technique 205
  X-rays 183
Adrenocorticotrophic hormone (ACTH), assay service 214
Age, maternal and Down's syndrome 25
AIDS
  blood transfusion 155
  hospital personnel risk 156
Amenorrhoea
  assessment 120, 121

Amenorrhoea (*cont.*)
  gonadotrophin therapy 144–7
  laboratory tests 120–3
Amniocentesis 5
  indications 29, 30
  procedure and timing 20
  uses 163
Anaemia; management 32, 62
Anaesthesia, *general*
    assessment 80, 81
    caesarian section 88, 89
    preparation 81
    risks 82
   .retained products evacuation 102
Analgesia *see also* epidural
  normal labour, first stage 54
    second stage 57
Anovulation 142
Antacids, first stage labour 54
Antenatal clinics 19–30
  agenda 23–6
  appointment timing 19–21
  booking 23
  design faults 23
  GP and hospital 21–3
  hospital 20, 21, 26
  improvements 19
  investigations 20
  origin and role 19
Antenatal wards
  admission, indications 31–4
  visiting 31
Antibiotics
  cardiac patients 170
  choice 168
  gynaecological surgery 190, 191
  intravenous additives 202
  prophylactic 167
Anticoagulant therapy
  dose and procedures 157, 158
  postoperative 195, 196
  prescribing 201
Anti-D 91
  rhesus haemolytic disease 158

Bed rest, definition *x*
Biparietal diameter, pregnancy chart 22
Birthplan, patients' own 26
Blood chemistry, reference ranges 159, 160
Blood cultures, instructions 166, 167
Blood products 156, 157
Blood sampling 49 *see also* fetal
  maternal cubital vein 49
  septic abortion 138
Blood transfusion 154–6
  cross-matching 154, 155
  emergency, safety 88
  hazards 155, 156
  uses 80
Bradycardia 43
Breast abscesses 168
Breast lumps 17
Breech delivery 67, 68
Bromocriptine 143
Buccal smear 133
  procedure 133, 134

Caesarian section
  anaesthesia 89
  closure 103, 105
  delivery 103, 104
  incision 103
  pre-medication 88, 89
  previous monitoring 62, 63
  RMO role 102
  and sterilization 102
  techniques 103
Calcitonin, assay service 214
Cancer
  ovarian, treatment protocol 175–9
    chart 176, 177
    dosage and administration 178, 179
  types, cytotoxic therapy 175
Carcinoembryonic antigen 174
  assay service 214
Cardiac sector scanner 15
Cardiotokography 22 *see also* fetal

Cardiovascular disorders 14–16
  antibiotic use 170
Catecholamines and renal function 164
Cervical intra-epithelial neoplasia (CIN) 150
  treatment and follow-up 152
Cervical smear, spatula 120, 121
Cervix
  annual suture 6
  carcinoma 17
  torn 69
Chest infection 170
Child abuse 28
Choriocarcinoma 174, 182
Chorion villus biopsy 5, 23, 24
  catheter, scheme 24
Clinical budgeting 207–9
  doctors' attitudes 208, 209
  financial systems 208
  ideas 207
  managements 207
Clinical chemistry 159–64
Clinics see also antenatal, postnatal
  antenatal 19–30
  postnatal 96
  pre-pregnancy 3
Clomiphene citrate and ovulation induction 143, 144
Colposcopy
  apparatus 150
  referral 150
  report form 151
Congenital infections 172
Consent forms 98
Contraception
  oral 93
  postnatal management 92–4
  use 26
Counselling 3
  clinics 4–6
  genetic 5
Creatinine clearance 164
Cryocautery 123, 124
  apparatus 124
Curettings, samples 195
Cyclophosphamide
  ovarian cancer therapy 175–9

Cyclophosphamide (*cont.*)
  side-effects 179
Cystitis, causes and treatment 169
Cytogenetic screening 121, 122
Cytotoxic therapy
  combination, ovarian cancer 175–9
  gynaecological cancers 175

Deep vein thrombosis 69
Delivery
  birthplan 27
  hospital 28
Diabetes mellitus 9–11
  maternal and fetal complications 11
  tests 10
Diet
  labour 54
  pre-pregnancy 4
Diploma of the Royal College of Obstetricians and Gynaecologists
    (DRCOG) 216
Down's syndrome and maternal age 25
Drugs
  controlled 201
  hazards 7
  intravenous additives 202
  monitoring 199
  route and dose 200
  use in pregnancy, 6, 7, 16
Dydrogesterone structure 130

Eclampsia management 62
Emergency *see also* flying squad
  gynaecological surgery 189
Endocrine testing 160–2 *see also* individual glands
Epidural analgesia 54
  bladder control 85
  blood pressure 84
  catheter removal 86
  cerebrospinal fluid tap 86
  complications 86, 87
  consent 83

Epidural analgesia (*cont.*)
   contraindications 82
   features 82
   local anaesthetic 83
   management and procedures 83–5
   second stage assessment 86
   top-ups 83, 84
Epilepsy 6, 7
Episiotomy 57
   alternatives' scheme 99, 100
Episiorrhaphy 57
   alternatives 99, 100
External cephalic version 65

Fellow of the Royal College of Surgeons (FRCS) 216
Ferritin assay 214
Fetal activity chart, Cardiff 36
Fetal blood sampling 45–9
   collection 48, 49
   electrodes 46
   endoscope 47, 48
   serial collections 47
   techniques 47–9
Fetal cardiotokography
   definitions 44, 45
   heart rate variation 41, 42
   intrapartum monitoring 44, 45
   terminology 43–5
   uses 37
Fetal distress, definition and management 64
Fetal heart rate
   acceleration 43–5
   deceleration 43–5
   descriptions 44
   and uterine contractions 45
   variability 41, 42, 44
Fetal kick chart 35
Fetal measurements, ultrasound 187, 188
Fetal monitoring 35–49 *see also* individual procedures
   antenatal 35–43
   indications 62, 63
   intrapartum 43–9
   investigations 49

Fetal pH 47
Fetal skin colour 48
Feto-placental function assessment 161, 162
α-Fetoprotein 25
  assay service 214
  assessment 26
    procedure 164
  maternal serum 30, 164
  neural defects 164
  tumour marker 174
Fetus, prostaglandin effects 67
Fibrinogen 157
Flying squad
  book 76
  calls, procedure 77, 78
  drugs 222
  equipment 77, 220, 221
  intravenous fluids 221
  practice runs 78
  registrar duties 78
  staff 76
Folic acid
  epileptic therapy 6, 7
  prophylactic 30
Forceps delivery 68

General practitioner obstetric units 73–8
  administration 75
  admission procedure 75, 76
  case selection 74, 75
  GP qualifications 73
  hospital staff role 74
  preparation 75
  responsibilities 73, 74
Genitourinary medicine 125–8
Gentamicin
  assay 172
  blood levels 171, 172
  indications 171
  and renal function 171, 172
Glucose tolerance test
  in diabetes 10
  procedure 163

Glycosylated haemoglobin (HbA$_1$) 10
Gonadotrophic releasing hormone, tests 123
Griffiths Report 207
Growth hormone, post-mortem extraction 225, 226
Gynaecological outpatients 119–28
   examination and investigations 119–23
   follow-up visits 125
   procedures 123–5

Haematinics 203–5
Haemorrhage
   antepartum, management 32, 64, 65
   intrapartum 64, 65
   postpartum, management 68
Heparin, gynaecological surgery 190
Hepatitis, serum; precautions and blood transfusion 156
High-risk pregnancy
   features 21
   GP units 75
   monitoring 75
Histopathology
   placental 152, 153
   request card 152
HLA antigens 134
Hospital
   discharge 94–6
      assessment 94, 95
   indications for admission 31–4
   readmission, indications 95, 96
Human chorionic gonadotrophin (HCG)
   levels, normal pregnancy 131
   ovulation induction 143, 144
      timing 145
   tumour markers 174
Human menopausal gonadotrophin (HMG)
   contraindications 145
   ovulation induction 144–6
Human placental lactogen (HPL)
   chart 40
   serial values and gestation 37, 39
Human Tissue Act 226
Husband, definition x

Hydatidiform mole
  chemotherapy 181
  diagnosis and management 139
  follow-up and pregnancy 181, 182
  registration 180
  tissue sampling 180
Hydroxyprogesterone caproate, structure 130
Hyperparathyroidism, management 14
Hypertension see also pregnancy-induced
  postpartum management 69
Hyperthyroidism, management 12, 13
Hypocalcaemic crisis 14
Hypopituitarism, management 12
Hypoparathyroidism, management 14
Hypothyroidism
  management 12
  transient 13
Hysterosalpingography 180

Immigrants, investigations 6
Immune defects, early pregnancy 134
Infertility 140–8
  endocrine investigations 162, 163
  female 142–8
    classification 146, 147
  gonadotrophin therapy 144–8
  investigations 140, 141
  male 141
  pituitary extracts 226
Intra-uterine death
  investigations 64
  management 64
Intravenous urogram 180
Investigations
  antenatal clinic 20, 23
  gynaecological 120
  infertility 140, 141, 162, 163
  postnatal 91
  pre-pregnancy 6
  recurrent abortion 133, 134
Iron see also total dose
  oral therapy 203
  preparations 203
  prophylactic 30

Karman curette 132
Ketosis 63

Labour
  abnormal, management 58–71
  birthplan 27
  feeding 81, 82
  induction techniques 66, 67
  monitoring records 55
  normal management 53–8
    first stage 53–6
    fourth stage 90 *see also* postnatal
    second stage 57
    third stage 58
  pre-term 58–60
    salbutamol infusion 59, 60
  supervision 55
Labour ward 51–71
  admission 51
  midwives 51
Laceration repair
  definition 99
  sutures 101
  third and fourth degree 99, 101
Lactation suppression 92
Laparoscopy, indications and morbidity 191
Leiofibromata 17
Luteinizing hormone-releasing hormone (LH-RH)
    ovulation induction 147
Lymphangiogram 186

Maternal distress 63
Maternal hypotension and epidural 87
Medical problems 9–14
    management 32
Medical profession and clinical budgeting 208, 209
Medical records 108
Medroxyprogesterone acetate, structure 130
Member of the Royal College of Physicians (MRCP) 216
Membranes
  premature rupture, management 33, 34

Membranes (*cont.*)
  rupture, precautions 66
Microbiology 165–73
Multiple pregnancy management 32, 33

Natural childbirth 67
Neonate
  heat loss prevention 113
  management 112
  maternal cross-infection 173
Neural tube defects 30
Nurses, training of male 228

Obstetric bed 52
Oestradiol 17-β, tests 123
Oestriol values 36, 37
  chart 38
  drugs affecting 35
  serial 161, 162
Oestrogens and gestation time 37
Oligohydramnios 63
Organs, transplantation 225
Ovarian antigen CX_1 assay 215
Ovulation induction
  drugs used 143–8
  investigations 142, 143
Oxytocin
  labour induction regime 66
  uses 55, 56, 71

Paediatrician, role and conditions 111, 112
Pain, abdominal 16
Papanicolau's smear, indications 149, 150
Partogram 56
Pathology requests 194, 195
Pelvic disorders 17, 25
Pelvic inflammatory disease
  investigations 167
  treatment 169

Perinatal mortality, diabetes 9
Perineal discomfort, ultrasound 92
Perineum breakdown 96
Phaeochromocytoma management 14
Pharmaceutical services 198–205
Pharmacist role 198
Pituitary disorders 12
Pituitary gonadotrophins, screening 122
Placenta
    alkaline phosphatase assay 215
    delivery, caesarian section 103, 104
    histology 153
    location 65
    retained, definition 70
        anaesthetists' role 88
        blood transfusion 80
        delivery procedure 70, 71
Placental function tests 22
    serial oestriol values 35, 36
Placentography 188
Postgraduate training courses 216–19
Postmortem examination
    certificate accuracy 224
    diagnosis accuracy 224
    educational use 224, 225
    permission 223
    reasons 223, 224
    request forms 226, 227
    therapeutic uses 225, 226
Postnatal clinic 96
Postnatal ward 90–6
    assessment and discharge 94, 95
    fourth stage 90
    haematological investigations 91
    microbiological investigations 91
Postoperative management 195–7
Potassium, intravenous additives 202, 203
Pre-eclampsia
    fulminating, monitoring 61, 62
    management and drugs 60, 61
Pregnancy, ectopic 139, 167
Pregnancy-induced hypertension *see also* eclampsia, pre-eclampsia
    management 32, 60–2
Pregnancy tests 121

Prescriptions
    alterations 200
    controlled drugs 201
    requirements 199–201
Pre-term *see* labour
Primigravida, elderly and young 62
Progesterone, structure 130
Progestogens, structures 130
Progestogen therapy, threatened abortion 129, 130
Prolactin screening 122
Prolactinoma management 12
Prolapsed cord management 71
Prostaglandins
    abortion 135, 136
    fetal roles 67
    labour induction 66, 67
    structures 137
Psychosexual problems 128
Psychotherapy 4
    intra-uterine death 64
    postoperative 195
Pudendal needle 84
Pulmonary embolism, management scheme 195, 196
Pyelonephritis
    causes and treatment 169, 170
    pregnancy 170
Pyrexia 91

Radiology 183–8
    preparation 185
    request cards 184
    safety and risk 183
    special procedures 185, 186
    ten-day rule 183
    ward 184, 185
Renal function tests 164
Resident medical officer (RMO)
    paediatrician and newborn 113
    records 108
    surgical competence 98
Respiratory paralysis and epidural 87
Resuscitation, newborn 112

Retained products, evacuation procedures 101, 102
Rhesus haemolytic disease, management 158
Rheumatic heart disease, antibiotic cover 15, 16
Rubella assessment 23

Salbutamol in pre-term labour 59, 60
Screening tests
    diabetes 9, 10
    genetic abnormalities 25
Semen analysis 141
Sexually transmitted diseases 126
    non-specific 126
    and promiscuity 127
    special clinics 127
    specimen collection 128
Shared-care protocol 21–3
Shock 69
    treatment 205
Small-for-dates
    management 31
    monitoring 60
Social work 28, 29
Spalding's sign 64
Special care 29
Special care baby units 111–15
    hospital transfer 114
    indications for admission 113, 114
    neonatal management 112
    resuscitation 112
Specimen collection 165
    sexually transmitted disease 128
Staff, definition x
Sterilization
    postpartum 16
        and discussion 93, 94
        methods 106, 107
    tubal histology 194
    tubal rings and clips 106, 107
Stillbirths 229
Stress in pregnancy 28
Supraregional assay service 214, 215
Surgery, gynaecological 189–97
    complications 195

Surgery (*cont.*)
    daycase procedures 192
    emergencies 189, 193
    follow-up 197
    operation lists 193
    pathology requests 194, 195
    postoperative management 195–7
    preoperative preparation 190, 191
Surgical disorders 16, 17
Surgical procedures 98–108 *see also* individual procedures, laceration
Syntometrine, use in third stage 58

T_3 monitoring 160, 161
    and infertility 163
T_4 monitoring 160, 161
    and infertility 163
Tachycardia 43
Tears, repair 70
Termination *see also* abortion
    and previous conception 6
Thyroid function tests 160–2
    normal ranges 161
Thyroid gland disorders 12, 13
Thyroid stimulating hormone (TSH)
    testing and infertility 160, 161, 163
Total dose iron-dextran technique (TDI) 204, 205
    procedure 204
    reactions 205
Tubal division 106
Tubal ligation methods 106, 107
Tumour markers 174
Tuohy needle 85

Ultrasound screening 121
    abortion 133
    chorion villus sampling 24
    department 187, 188
    frequency 26
    gynaecological uses 187
    indications 10
    obstetric uses 187, 188

Ultrasound screening (*cont.*)
  pelvic organs 120
  retained products 101
  side effects 28
Ultrasound therapy, perineal 92
Urinary steroids, testing 122
Urinary tract infection, treatment 169, 170
Urine specimens 165
Urofollitrophin and ovulation induction 147, 148
Uterine contraction
  pressure and duration 43
  suppression 59, 60

Vaccination, rubella 7, 91
Vagina, infection; causes and treatment 169
Vaginal swabs 165, 166
Venereal disease *see also* sexually transmitted disease
  use of term 127
Vitamin D analogue 14
Vitamin supplementation 7

Warfarin use and age 157, 158
Weight
  conversion chart 213
  normal and accepted 5
Wound infections 166, 168, 169
  treatments 168

X-ray departments 183 *see also* radiology